First Steps in Clinical Supervision

A guide for healthcare professionals

First Steps in Clinical Supervision

Supervision

A guide for healthcare professionals

Paul Cassedy

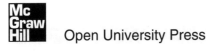
Open University Press

Open University Press
McGraw-Hill Education
McGraw-Hill House
Shoppenhangers Road
Maidenhead
Berkshire
England
SL6 2QL

email: enquiries@openup.co.uk
world wide web: www.openup.co.uk

and Two Penn Plaza, New York, NY 10121-2289, USA

First published 2010

A catalogue record of this book is available from the British Library

ISBN 978 0 33523 651 0 (pb) 978 033523 650 3 (hb)
ISBN 10: 0335236510 (pb) 0335236502 (hb)

Library of Congress Cataloging-in-Publication Data
CIP data applied for

Typeset by RefineCatch Limited, Bungay, Suffolk
Printed in the UK by Bell & Bain Ltd, Glasgow

Mixed Sources
Product group from well-managed
forests and other controlled sources
www.fsc.org Cert no. TT-COC-002769
© 1996 Forest Stewardship Council

The *McGraw·Hill* Companies

This book is dedicated to my Mum and Dad who always give me love, guidance and quality care.

Also to my sons and daughter, Daniel, Jackson, Phoebe and Jake, who give me continuous learning.

In loving memory of my brother, Martin, who was always there for me when needed.

Gratitude is not only the greatest of virtues, but the parent of all others.
—Cicero (106–43 BC)

Contents

Acknowledgements   x
List of figures   xi

1 Introducing Clinical Supervision   1

   Introduction   2
   Are similar roles already in place?   2
   Reaching a definition   3
   Some background information   5
   This supervisor's background   6
   The name of clinical supervision   7
   Supervision as a journey   8
   Is supervision therapy?   8
   Categorizing clinical supervision into functions   10
   Benefits of clinical supervision   13
   What are the reasons for becoming a supervisor?   15
   Relevant collaboration with others   19
   Training for clinical supervision   21
   Conclusion   22

2 What to Cover at a First Meeting   24

   Introduction   24
   The purpose of a supervision contract   25
   Essential elements of a supervision contract   26
   Negotiation of rights and responsibilities   26
   Making contributions to the supervision relationship   29
   Putting in a little extra   31
   Getting started with the first meeting   32
   What has brought us here? Expectations for supervision   33
   Contracting for supervision: agreeing the practicalities   36
   Note taking and record keeping   37
   Introducing and making a contract   40
   Conclusion   43

3 Qualities for a Healthy Supervision Relationship   45

   Introduction   45

The essence of a supervision relationship 46
Characteristics of a supervision relationship 47
Person-centred theory 48
The core conditions of helping and the supervision relationship 49
Self-awareness and the clinical supervisor 55
A self-awareness framework 57
Giving constructive feedback 61
Conclusion 65

4 Three Functions of Clinical Supervision 67

Introduction 67
The normative function 70
The formative function 72
The restorative function 74
A balance of support and challenge 79
Changing supervisors 82
The three functions and research 83
Conclusion 84

5 Active Listening and Responding Skills 85

Introduction 85
Listening as a supervisor 86
Core principles for effective listening in supervision 88
Non-verbal communication and listening 89
Combining non-verbal cues with the spoken word 91
Perceiving non-verbal communication 92
Getting ready to listen 94
The supervisor's toolbox of active listening skills 94
Conclusion 105

6 Six-Category Intervention Analysis 106

Introduction 106
The value of six-category intervention analysis to the
    clinical supervisor 107
The prescriptive category 110
The informative category 113
The confronting category 115
The cathartic category 118
The catalytic category 120
The supportive category 121
Six-category intervention analysis for clinical supervision 123
The need to be aware of degenerative interventions 126
Conclusion 128

7 A Problem-Solving Framework: The Skilled Helper Model   129

Introduction   129
Reasons for a problem-solving model   131
Stage 1. The current scenario or problem situation   134
Stage 2. The preferred scenario   140
Stage 3. Action strategies   145
Some final thoughts   149
Conclusion   150

8 Reflective Practice and the Supervisor   152

Introduction   152
Defining reflective practice   153
Reflective practice in clinical supervision   154
Reasons for a reflective framework   156
A model of reflection   156
Using reflective cycles and models together   161
Conclusion   162
Suggested further reading   162

9 Structuring and Evaluating Clinical Supervision Sessions   163

Introduction   163
Does a session need a framework?   165
Which framework to choose?   166
A simple format   167
Interpersonal process recall   173
Self-assessment checklist for clinical supervisors   175
Evaluation in clinical supervision   178
When clinical supervision comes to an end   181
Conclusion   182

10 Avoiding Stress and Burnout as a Supervisor   183

Introduction   183
Stress and burnout   184
Taking care of yourself   187
The spirit of supervision   188
Some ways to combat stress and replenish yourself   189
Who supervises the supervisor?   190
Conclusion   191

References   193
Index   199

Acknowledgements

I would like to thank all those involved at Open University Press who have contributed to the production of this book, especially Rachel Crookes who was brave enough to support me following the first draft and offered valuable guidance and suggestions.

I thank my friends and colleagues at the School of Nursing, Nottingham University ,who have given encouragement and support in a variety of ways. In particular I would like to mention Trish Bateman, Andrew Clifton, Ada Hui, Jane McGregor, Nigel Plant, Lorraine Rayner and Dave Wilson.

I acknowledge and thank all the supervisors and supervisees I have had the privilege of working with over the years, without whom I would not have been in any position to write this book.

I also thank with much gratitude all my friends , who know who they are but they like to remain anonymous, for helping me do something that I could not have done alone.

List of figures

1.1   Triangle for supervision implementation   20
2.1   Example sheet for recording clinical supervision content   39
3.1   The Johari Window   57
3.2   Johari Window applied to supervision   59
4.1   A conceptual framework for clinical supervision   68
4.2   Supervisor style of normative interventions   70
4.3   A balance of support and challenge   80
6.1   Heron's six-category intervention analysis   108
6.2   Six-category intervention analysis applied to clinical supervision   109
7.1   The skilled helper model   132
7.2   Stage 1: the current scenario   134
7.3   Stage 2: the preferred scenario   141
7.4   Stage 3: action strategies   146
7.5   Force field analysis   148
8.1   A reflective cycle   157
9.1   A reflective cycle for developing supervision competences   179
9.2   Evaluation of clinical supervision sessions   180

1

Introducing Clinical Supervision

Chapter outcomes

By reading this chapter, doing the reflective activities, and integrating the material into your supervision practice, you should be able to:

- Acknowledge the difference between clinical supervision and similar roles already in practice.
- Understand a definition of clinical supervision.
- Know some background information to the emergence of clinical supervision.
- Acknowledge the difference between clinical supervision and therapy.
- Gain an overview of the functions of clinical supervision.
- Become aware of the main benefits of clinical supervision.
- Recognize and reflect on transferable skills which can assist becoming a supervisor.
- Recognize the importance of having guidelines for the introduction of clinical supervision.
- Recognize the importance and value of collaboration when implementing the guidelines of clinical supervision.
- Acknowledge the value of a training programme and know what to look for.

Introduction

Welcome to *First Steps in Clinical Supervision*. The words 'clinical supervision' are now known to the majority of people working in the helping professions but there still may be some misunderstanding of the concept. This first chapter offers a broad overview and introduction to clinical supervision, focusing on what I believe a beginning supervisor needs to know and have understanding of. I hope it will also begin to clarify any misunderstandings you may have and raise issues and questions you may want to discuss. The chapter focuses on some of the important concepts, information and related issues that will be valuable to you as you take your first steps to becoming a clinical supervisor.

Becoming a clinical supervisor can be a rewarding yet challenging experience for the healthcare professional. I am assuming that, having picked up this book, you are in a position to take on the role of supervisor or are already in that role. You want to acquire more knowledge and skills and to further your understanding and development. You may need to remind yourself, as I still often do, of some of the pitfalls that we can slip into. You may need to revise existing skills or to have a look at and practise some new ones. Whatever your need, I hope you find something of interest here that will help you to reflect on your role and work as a supervisor. I hope you can go on to enjoy your role as supervisor and become good, and then great, at what you do: don't just settle for being good enough. Aim high. Read more on the subject, develop more by continuing to reflect on your supervision practice, seek feedback from your supervisees and relevant others who are involved in the implementing process, and seek out further training and updates. Becoming proactive in this role will help you to lay the foundations upon which you can build towards your goals of increasing your potential and enabling quality practice as a supervisor.

Supervision is about working with people. Therefore you will be able to draw upon the many interpersonal and communication skills you use in your various roles in clinical practice. You may already have been involved in a role similar to that of a clinical supervisor, and, for some, this may be where a misunderstanding of the clinical supervisor's role arises. I aim to address this in the next section.

Are similar roles already in place?

Several formal and informal professional roles are already in place that can serve some of the different functions of supervision. These roles will be fulfilled by such people as line managers, mentors, preceptors, tutors, consultant specialists and colleagues. Many other support systems are, however, time limited and have a specific focus and serve a specific need. For example, a newly qualified nurse is given a preceptor for 6 to 12 months, student nurses are allocated a mentor, staff support groups are arranged for debriefing sessions. Wilson (2000) purports that to distinguish between similar roles and clinical supervision can be a *'thorny problem'* (p. 187) as at times those roles have been interchangeable and there is inconsistency among the terms used and their prescribed uses. He goes on to consider the differences to good effect and puts a strong case for the defined role of clinical supervision. Lynch et al. (2008) also comprehensively distinguish clinical supervision from other formal relationships and examine some common myths and misconceptions. Scaife (2009) explores how the term 'clinical supervision' has been used in the literature, detailing the features that characterize supervision and that help to distinguish it from similar activities.

If there is an answer to the question 'are similar roles already in place?', it is not an entirely obvious one, and therein lies the conundrum. However, my answer would be as follows:

> Other, similar roles may serve some of the functions of clinical supervision some of the time, but not all of the functions of clinical supervision all of the time.

I believe that the role of the clinical supervisor is to merge aspects of the similar roles. But in doing so, the clinical supervisor is forming a distinct and formal regular relationship for the purpose of and aim of clinical supervision. Supervision is therefore designed for career lifelong enhancement of clinical practice, support and learning, for all healthcare staff. It becomes a unique and tailor-made relationship for the supervisee, where they feel safe and supported enough to reflect and learn while exploring their clinical practice to enhance patient and client care.

Reaching a definition

As clinical supervision began to emerge across the healthcare professions, Butterworth and Faugier (1992) acknowledged the difficulty in reaching a precise definition of the term. As the seeds of ideas have been planted, so numerous definitions of clinical supervision have seen the light of day in the increasing number of books and papers on the subject. These definitions reflect to some extent the scope of the term as there is a diversity of healthcare settings where it is being implemented and of practitioners to whom it is being applied.

As the supervision relationship is the vehicle for its success, a definition also needs to reflect on the relationship between supervisor and supervisee. Faugier (1992) outlines this well. She proposes the essential characteristics and espouses the qualities of a supervision relationship. Definitions of supervision may differ across different healthcare settings and groups, but a review of the literature reveals three general areas for practice:

- Quality assurance and the provision of quality care and standards.
- A method of learning to develop and improve practice.
- Professional and personal support.

Brockelhurst (1994) identified common features in numerous definitions of clinical supervision which encompass the above, managerial, educational and supportive, elements:

- Supervision is an active process necessitating equal input from supervisor and supervisee.
- The process of supervision requires structures and procedures.
- Supervision has a number of related aims: ensuring safe practice, developing skills, encouraging personal and professional growth, and supporting staff.
- The supervision relationship is of fundamental importance.

Note the following definitions which incorporate those terms:

> *A formal process of professional support and learning which enables individual practitioners to develop knowledge and competence, assume responsibility for their own practice, and enhance consumer protection and the safety of care in complex clinical situations.*
>
> (Department of Health 1993)

> *As a working alliance between practitioners in which they aim to enhance clinical practice ... [to] meet ethical, professional and best practice standards. While providing personal support and encouragement in relation to professional practice ...*
>
> (Kavanagh et al. 2002: 247)

It is interesting to note that the latter and more recent definition includes the term 'working alliance', to emphasize the importance and value of the supervision relationship. A review by Kilminster and Jolly (2000) concludes that *'the quality of the supervision relationship is probably the single most important factor for the effectiveness of supervision'*. Borders (2005) also identifies that the supervisor–supervisee relationship is critical to the overall process.

A working alliance can be defined in this context as a working partnership based on a mutual agreement to fulfil the expectations of clinical supervision. This, now often referred to as a supervisory alliance, will require of the supervisor such qualities as will enable them to establish a trusting and empathic relationship. The skills to develop a safe and facilitative learning climate are also required.

In my definition that follows, and the one I shall be working with, I have importantly included the words 'facilitation' and 'relationship' to emphasize how the three main functions of support, learning and quality care can be enhanced.

> Clinical supervision can be defined as a regular and formal agreement to engage in a professional working relationship, facilitated by the supervisor to support the supervisee to reflect on practice, with the aim of developing quality care, accountability, personal competence and learning.

Reflective activity

Drawing on your own understanding and experience of clinical supervision as they are now, ask yourself:

- What is important for you to include in a definition of clinical supervision?
- How do your fellow healthcare professionals define clinical supervision?
- Do you feel the definition and objectives of supervision are up for debate? If not why not?
- How are you going to define what clinical supervision is when asked by a colleague or a new supervisee?

Some background information

Clinical supervision began to appear in the 1920s in classical psychoanalysis. The concept developed and became integrated into the practice of professions using psychotherapeutic forms of treatment. Reference can be found in the literature of psychotherapy, counselling, psychology, psychiatry, social work and occupational therapy.

Hildegard Peplau (1909–1999) was influential in helping to give prominence to the practice of supervision in nursing. The subject has been appearing in literature for healthcare professionals in the United Kingdom since the 1980s, and in 1982 the Registered Mental Nurse syllabus flagged up the term 'clinical supervision'. The Department of Health report *A Vision for the Future* (1993) included the following key target related specifically to clinical supervision:

The concept of clinical supervision should be further explored and developed. Discussion should be held at local and national level on the range and appropriateness of clinical supervision and a report made to the professionals.

Since that time the concept has been debated, recommended and advocated by healthcare academics, educationalists, managers and practitioners throughout the United Kingdom. During the 1990s, clinical supervision became better established and was recommended for practice across all the helping professions (Butterworth and Faugier 1992; Hawkins and Shohet 2000). The factors that created this drive derived from the many political, professional, educational and managerial changes that were taking place in healthcare delivery. Fowler (1996), Bond and Holland (1998) and Driscoll (2000) offer more detailed accounts of the emergence and developments of clinical supervision for healthcare practice.

This supervisor's background

My own nursing background was in mental health. It was when I was a community psychiatric nurse that, as a team, we started a support group among ourselves which took on some of the elements of clinical supervision. I was at the time undertaking a counselling skills certificate, and supervision was a fundamental part to the training. I began to recognize the importance of support when in the role of helper, and learnt the values of exploring oneself in relation to client work and efficacy of practice. Further training in humanistic psychology brought me into contact with a variety of practitioners and trainers, all of whom I have learnt something from in the vast arena of therapeutic growth and development. I moved into nurse education, where I was able to pass on some of that experience and knowledge on the various interpersonal skills training courses that I was involved in.

I continued my counselling practice and was fortunate to receive both group and individual supervision from a variety of supervisors. Increasingly over the years I have reaped the benefits – and I believe my clients have too – of supervision, as I have developed personally and professionally and become more effective and therapeutic as a counsellor. Further studies in counselling practice enabled me to explore more academically the role and function of supervision while assimilating and synthesizing the theories and concepts.

I have subsequently been involved in various aspects of supervision for many years. I have been a supervisor to various healthcare staff before the practice became fully established within their organizations. I facilitate group supervision and, through attending training courses, workshops and conferences, I have helped develop and deliver training programmes for clinical supervision within my role as a tutor. I have also facilitated others to help implement supervision in their practice settings and I supervise supervisors.

Few, if any, of the materials, theories and frameworks in this book are new ideas or approaches in the arena of supervision, interpersonal skills and personal development. I have merged some concepts and adapted them to a clinical supervision context. I have also integrated many of the skills and ideas that supervisors and educators have used with me in the past, utilizing and learning from the most helpful as well as the least helpful. They have been accumulated, tried and tested over time, and there is still ongoing development within my training and supervision practice. I adhere to a statement made by Shohet (1985), that we teach what we most need to learn. That phrase has lived with me over time, and as the years have passed I am still learning my trade. I only hope that, to rephrase a lesson from the Dalai Lama which is pertinent here, in my older years I can look back with some pride and a little honour on the work I have been involved in, so through those memories I might be able to enjoy those experiences a second time. If that hope is to come to fruition, I firmly believe that the supervision I have myself experienced will have been essential in enabling the work of which I am proud.

One reason that I introduced myself like this is that you, as a supervisor, will probably be called upon when starting your role to say something of yourself, your background and your experience – but probably not, I hope, all in one go as I have here.

The name of clinical supervision

From my experience of delivering training in supervision I am aware that the word 'supervision' conjures up a variety of thoughts and feelings. These thoughts have resulted from practitioners' prior experiences and opinions, both positive and negative. Both confusion and cynicism have had a direct influence on levels of enthusiasm and interest in the subject. It has also been suggested that the term 'clinical supervision' is a rather unfavourable one. It can conjure up images of the superintendent on surveillance duty. The made up word of 'snoopervision' I have also heard voiced. Yet, if you look up the two words 'clinical' and 'supervisor' in the dictionary you will find a supervisor described as an 'overseer' and clinical as 'observation of the patient'. I find the term perfectly adequate for the purpose and functions. 'Reflective practice' has been suggested as a more favourable term, but I feel this does not fully meet the functions and aims of clinical supervision.

Try dissecting the word so it becomes 'super – vision', as this perhaps highlights that it is not as prescriptive as it at first seems. The aim is to create a process where the supervisee can have access to and increase a super form of vision over their work and performance. For the purposes of this book, the term 'supervision' will be used when referring to what is generally agreed to be 'clinical supervision'.

Reflective activity

- Reflect on the words 'clinical supervision'.
- Be aware of your own experience in the past, when someone has been 'overseeing' you in relation to patient care.
- How have those experiences influenced your current conception of the term 'clinical supervision'?
- Would you consider modifying the name? If so, what to?
- How are you going to describe and define the title of 'clinical supervisor'?

Supervision as a journey

The metaphor of a journey has been used to describe the developmental process of supervision for both of the parties involved. I also subscribe to that notion, and supervision has for me been about exploration and discovery. As a supervisor, however, we must be clear that it is our supervisee's journey that we are now working on and that this journey is to be continuous. I hope by reading this book you may find, explore and discover ideas, techniques and thoughts that will assist you with the task and opportunity in front of you. It is a privilege to be a supervisor as you are entering into a unique learning journey with your supervisee. It is an opportunity to build a relationship on trust and honesty and one that embodies professional and personal development for the overall aim of enhancing healthcare practice.

Is supervision therapy?

If supervision is a journey and a developmental process, it is necessary to clarify the boundary between supportive supervision and therapy, as this can be problematic. You will need to ask yourself where the boundary between supervision and counselling lies. This question can surface when the supervisee is under stress as a result of the often emotionally draining and challenging work they are carrying out. You will need to consider, for example, if the source of stress is current personal or professional relationships and issues, or whether it is more personal to the supervisee and more deeply rooted in their past. These deeply rooted problems, that still surface, are often referred to in therapy as 'family of origin' experiences and certainly would not be an area to focus on. Whatever the causes of current stress and strain, you will need to ask yourself why you might need to pursue them and whether this should be focused on in supervision.

To begin to address the question of 'is supervision therapy?', I agree with Bernard and Goodyear (1998: 7) who recommend that *'any therapeutic intervention with supervisees . . . should only be in the service of helping supervisees become more effective with clients'*. They go on to state that providing therapy that has more comprehensive intentions is ethical misconduct. Scaife (2001) also notes there is a clear distinction between therapy and supervision in terms of the former being learning for life, and the latter learning for work.

There are inevitably some similarities between supervision and counselling. Skills of active listening and qualities of developing a working alliance are common to both. The environment and arrangements may also be similar. Regular sessions are arranged by formal mutual agreement, and the sessions take place in private. As a supervisor you need to be aware of these similarities, as the supervisees may at first have apprehensions and anxieties that perhaps supervision is counselling. You need to be clear of your role, not just in being able to define it but also in being able to distinguish it from counselling. You need to be able to discuss and explore the parameters and be clear in your own mind where the boundaries are and when you are straying from the task of supervision. Scaife (2009: 17) suggests that it is always useful for the supervisor to have in mind the question *'how is it relevant to the work?'* as a means of preserving the boundary between supervision and therapy. However, your counselling skills can be utilized as and when appropriate during sessions. You may want to think of it as work therapy when you are using counselling skills for supportive intentions. Always have in mind, though, that your therapeutic interventions are for the benefit, first and foremost, of the supervisee's performance and ability to practise effectively in their work setting and organization. Consider, for example, a situation in which your supervisee has recently suffered the loss of a parent due to a recurring illness. They have returned to work but do not feel quite 'back on their feet again', and they still have mixed or unfamiliar emotions that are at times affecting their concentration. You need to be supportive and to utilize counselling skills in enabling the supervisee to regain personal and professional ability and personal confidence. But what if that parent had an unexpected or tragic death and has left your supervisee in shock, and they have returned to work to try to get on with things and cope? You need to ask yourself whether you are competent and skilled enough to help support them through their recent trauma and whether supervision is the appropriate place for this. You need also to recognize, as they may not be aware of this themself, that they would benefit from further and more specialist expertise.

To summarize, here are some important points to consider:

- Clinical supervision is not personal counselling or therapy.
- Counselling skills can be utilized in supervision to provide support with the focus clearly on the supervisee's performance, ability and effectiveness in their work setting.

- As a supervisor, I have the necessary skills, knowledge and confidence to provide this support.
- As a supervisor, I have the awareness to suggest to the supervisee that perhaps they might seek more professional help and experience.
- As a supervisor, I am able to recognize and advise the supervisee that they do require further professional help.
- As a supervisor, I am aware of the resources and services available to the supervisee for any further professional help and support.

Categorizing clinical supervision into functions

The concept of clinical supervision accommodates a wide berth within a wide range of helping organizations. There also is a vast amount of literature that examines the many contexts that clinical supervision serves. Nevertheless, even within those different environments, supervision follows and endorses similar aims and objectives as well as guidelines and principles. Funnelling the various aims and functions into a coherent structure that became workable for healthcare professionals was a task to be achieved. It was from Kadushin's (1992) original framework that Proctor (1986) put forward a categorization of supervision that would help identify the functions and components of clinical supervision in healthcare settings today.

Proctor's (1986) three categories are:

- Normative (managerial)
- Formative (learning/educational)
- Restorative (supportive)

I have identified in brackets the functions that the category serves, but if you have not done so already, familiarize yourself with the terms 'normative', 'formative' and 'restorative'. They can be referred to as both categories and functions.

Many authors, for example Bond and Holland (1998), Power (1999) and Driscoll (2000), refer to the three categories as main functions of clinical supervision and advocate them as a framework for the supervisor and organizations to adopt. Many organizational policy statements on clinical supervision in the United Kingdom now cite these three functions in the context of a framework as a focus to meet aims and objectives of supervision. I strongly support those views, as this framework is particularly suited to healthcare settings as it focuses on tasks and roles (Inskipp and Proctor 1993).

As well as being a conceptual framework for the aims and objectives of supervision, the normative, formative and restorative categories can also help to identify a focus for the following:

- The qualities, skills and knowledge of a clinical supervisor.
- A training programme for clinical supervisors.
- The anticipated benefits of clinical supervision.
- A focus for evaluation and research.

Let us now take a brief look at the normative, formative and restorative categories and the key functions they serve for clinical supervision.

A managerial category – normative

- This function of clinical supervision is concerned with maintaining and developing standards of safe, ethical and quality practice.
- The focus is on enhancing the effectiveness and ability of the supervisee's clinical role and performance for and within the organization.

As a clinical supervisor you are helping the supervisee to examine and reflect on the work they do and explore ways of maintaining and improving quality and efficiency for the good and care of the patient. Supervision provides an opportunity to reflect on complex cases and issues. Individual thoughts and feelings regarding approaches to treatment, care, evaluation and planning can be reflected upon in clinical discussions that take place within the clinical environment. Such discussions provide an opportunity to demonstrate accountability and responsibility in the continuous improvement for practice (UKCC 1996; NMC 2005a). The normative category is in place also to ensure national and clinical guidelines are adhered to and the supervisee is working to those objectives.

Clinical supervision, however, is not line management: for example there is no role for formal appraisal of performance, and you are not in this role as the supervisee's manager. However, as supervisor you are often wearing a managerial hat regarding the above issues, as you may need to raise matters of concern, and respond and make any decisions with the supervisee as appropriate. Ideally, a clinical supervisor will not be the supervisee's line manager as this may result in a conflict and confusion of roles. A line manager will also have certain administrative duties that they need to fulfil which may preclude a supervision relationship with a member of their own staff. This, however, does not mean that a line manager is unable to be a clinical supervisor. If they have the skills and self-awareness to be a clinical supervisor it may not be their title that is the issue so much as their other roles and responsibilities in relation to their supervisee.

A learning and educative category – formative

- This function of clinical supervision is to help you to reflect with confidence on your professional role, knowledge and skills as an individual and within a multidisciplinary team.

- The focus is to enable you to learn and develop professional skills by receiving feedback and to develop new ideas.

This category assists the supervisee to become aware of strengths and weaknesses in their work. By developing insight through reflective practice and becoming more knowledgeable, the supervisee can relate theory to practice and integrate this learning in their clinical practice. This may lead to identification of specific training and development needs. However, as a supervisor you must remember that you are not the supervisee's tutor or teacher, although at times you may be wearing those hats.

A supportive category – restorative

- This function of clinical supervision is concerned with how the supervisee responds emotionally to the stresses of working in a helping environment and caring for others, while allowing time for self-appraisal and well-being.
- The focus is on building a nurturing supportive relationship that can help reduce stress while providing motivation and encouragement.

Helping your supervisee express feelings and concerns as an individual in their work can also help in developing insights into and new perspectives on ways to manage. Hawkins and Shohet (2000) refer to this category as 'pit head time': *'The right to wash off the grime of the work in the boss's time, rather than take it home'* (p. 51).

This protected and planned time is also a time to balance up the positive aspects by encouragement, praise and constructive feedback. However, remember that while in this role you are not the supervisee's counsellor, although you will be utilizing counselling skills as and when appropriate.

The many factors and issues that arise in each of the three categories are integrated and feed into each other. To develop the skills of being a clinical supervisor, therefore, will require flexibility, creativity and knowledge of individual supervisees' needs and experience. The normative, formative and restorative functions are explored in more depth in Chapter 4, where consideration is given to the skills needed for the supervisor.

Reflective activity

Consider and reflect on the normative, formative and restorative functions that have been described.

- Has your experience of clinical supervision included elements of each of the functions?
- If not, why not? (This could be because you receive different types of supervision, e.g. caseload and managerial supervision from your manager.)

- Do you feel there are any objectives of supervision that would no place within those three categories?
- What would be your case for that objective? Would other supervisors ag. with you?

Benefits of clinical supervision

Before we move on to explore some of your reasons for becoming a supervisor, I will make a list of the possible benefits that clinical supervision can have. Research-based evidence is still rather thin on the ground, and Cutcliffe (2001) argues that to link improved patient care with received clinical supervision is extremely problematic to orchestrate. If clinical supervision is to be firmly established in this millennium and sustained, there is a need for more rigorous research, in particular studies on the effectiveness of clinical supervision with patient or client outcomes. Rafferty et al. (2007: 233) poignantly point out that '*this remains the Holy Grail for clinical supervision research*'. The benefits to nurses of clinical supervision are, however, evident in several studies, and there is an overwhelming positive response (Butterworth et al. 1997). Some of the positive outcomes demonstrated by these studies are:

- Improved worker retention (Harvey and Schramski 1984).
- Maintenance of clinical skills and quality practice (Webb 1997).
- Improved communication among workers (Webb 1997).
- Increased job satisfaction (Butterworth et al. 1997; Milne and Westerman 2001).
- Support for supervisees in a regular and formal arrangement to discuss clinical practice (Teasdale et al. 2001).

The following set of outcomes can be described as anticipated benefits of good quality clinical supervision. I have grouped them under the headings of normative, formative and restorative and whom they could possibly benefit.

Normative function: benefiting the organization
- Safeguards standards of patient care by promoting best practice.
- Promotes self-awareness of professional accountability.
- Committed staff because they work in a culture where learning and development are valued.
- A culture in which work is valued and patients are valued.
- Staff have the opportunity to be proactive as the organization is more flexible and creative.

- Encourages patient-focused care as planning and care options are reflected on.
- Provides a sounding board for decision making.
- Reduction in sickness rates.
- More likely to retain and recruit staff.

Formative function: benefiting the supervisee

- Learning opportunities for both supervisee and supervisor.
- Promotes integration of learning and practice.
- Encourages and supports lifelong learning.
- Encourages reflective practice on performance, efficacy and development of analytical skills.
- Increased self-awareness on aspects of work-related personal and professional responsibilities and abilities.
- Helps to identify further training and educational needs for personal and professional development.

Restorative function: benefiting the supervisee

- Support for emotional release.
- Validation and affirmation of ideas, views and feelings.
- Challenge and feedback on current thinking leading to new understanding and development.
- Increased motivation.
- Increased creativity.
- Increased staff support and morale.

Benefiting the patient

- All of the above.
- Empathic nursing care.
- Motivated nursing care.
- Ethical-based nursing care.

Most, if not all, of the above would integrate and correlate with each other. I need to emphasize again that the above are only what can be described as the possible or anticipated outcomes and benefits. I have based this on the supervision literature I have read, also on my observations and understandings by listening, and on discussions in my practice and teaching of clinical supervision. I have suggested in Chapter 9 that some of the above would be possible to consider when it comes to evaluating supervision, for example themes and key areas that the supervisee brings to supervision and the perceived outcomes. For those of you who want to further investigate research methods that have been developed for clinical supervision, I suggest Gilmore (2001) and Winstanley (2001).

What are the reasons for becoming a supervisor?

Fitzgerald (2000) and Faugier (1992) are among many writers who have detailed some of the attributes and skills you need to become a supervisor. Some of these qualities you may already have in your locker and they will help and enable you on your journey. When considering reasons for becoming a supervisor I will again use the headings from the three categories of clinical supervision that describe its aims and purposes. I have adapted from Driscoll (2000) the following transferable skills as they are good indicators of what may possibly help and be needed for the role. I suggest you consider the following reasons and skills as you take your first steps towards becoming a clinical supervisor. Your confidence should benefit if you have experience of or are involved in some of the activities and situations mentioned.

Managerial reasons for becoming a supervisor (normative)

- You have asked to be a clinical supervisor following the various initiatives and policies that are now being implemented in your place of work.
- You have taken the initiative yourself.
- You are a firm believer in clinical supervision.
- You want to transfer existing skills you have in similar roles, into a more formal and defined role of clinical supervisor.

Examples of skills that would transfer into the normative role

- Being knowledgeable about organizational guidelines and policies relating to patient safety and codes of conduct.
- You have some knowledge and understanding of ethical standards that underpin your professional work.
- You have handled complaints with diplomacy.
- You participate in multidisciplinary team meetings and liaise with other healthcare professionals.
- You have completed objectives set at your last appraisal or personal review.
- You have had experience of managing within your clinical area and team.
- You have been called upon to express your professional opinion from senior colleagues.
- You have at times challenged more senior colleagues when standards and quality of care have been an issue.
- You are knowledgeable regarding the NMC professional code of conduct (2008) and related statutory issues, for example those regarding confidentially in clinical supervision.
- You are comfortable in the role of authority.
- You have experience of your own clinical supervision.

Reflective activity

- Make a note of which of the above skills and abilities you may need to experience or enhance.
- What other activities or roles would it be possible for you to adopt?
- Add any additional transferable skills that you have.
- How comfortable are you with the perceived position of authority and the actual responsibility that you have as supervisor?

Power and authority

When you occupy the position of supervisor you may be perceived to be in a powerful and authoritative role. This power may also be derived from being an expert in your field. This, however, should not be an encouragement to fall into the trap of seeing the supervisee as powerless. Whenever possible and plausible, involve the supervisee in the important decision making and problem solving. Such interventions also promote relationship building and working together. This might be achieved by saying something along the lines of, 'I am wondering what you think would be the best way to take this forward?' or, 'Would it be okay if I paused for a moment there? You are asking many significant questions and it's important for you that we come up with some suitable ideas. What are your first thoughts?'

There may very well be issues on which you do need to exert your authority. Among these will be when you need to refer to the supervision contract, issues regarding the professional code of conduct and other issues of concern regarding your supervisee. These are considered and explored more in Chapter 2.

Learning reasons for becoming a supervisor (formative)

- To further develop your knowledge and skills in the area of clinical practice.
- To further your skills and development as a trainer and educator.
- To become more creative in your role.

Examples of skills that would transfer into the formative role

- You have experience of working as a preceptor.
- You have experience of teaching junior members of staff.
- You subscribe to a relevant practice journal.
- You worked as part of a team and contributed to a relevant research project.
- You have attended study days or training in clinical supervision.
- You have experience of your own clinical supervision.

Reflective activity

- Make a note of which of the above skills and abilities you may need to experience or enhance.
- What other activities or roles would it be possible for you to adopt?
- Add any additional transferable skills and abilities that you have.

Supportive reasons for becoming a clinical supervisor (restorative)

- You are able to recognize and acknowledge that you are a good listener.
- Others tend to come to you to talk and open up more about themselves regarding patient care, work issues, or just to offload in general.
- You are able to recognize when something is bothering you and are able to confide in someone you trust.

Examples of skills that would transfer into the restorative role

- You demonstrate when appropriate the need for teamworking and bonding.
- Feedback from student evaluations cites your supportive and welcoming approach.
- You have experience of being a member of a support group.
- You have experience of being a patient's advocate.
- You have experience of your own clinical supervision.

Reflective activity

- Make a note of which of the above skills and abilities you may need to experience or enhance.
- What other activities or roles would it be possible for you to adopt?
- Add any additional transferable skills and abilities that you have.
- In what situations in your work role do you feel helpless?
- Who will support you?

In the past, most supervisors in healthcare settings would have been placed in that position because of their experience with clinical skills and because their current position of responsibility enabled them to take on the role (Campbell 2006). However, becoming a supervisor and to be effective in the role demands additional knowledge, skills and abilities. It is also a responsible and senior position, and you need to be sure you are comfortable with the role. It is important that you have not been pressured or forced into this role as you may then struggle with the level of commitment that is going to be needed. As a clinical supervisor you also need experience of clinical supervision. Kohner (1994) and Rolfe et al. (2001) state not only that the supervisor should have training but also that they should be in a supervision relationship on their own behalf.

You need to be genuine and honest with yourself in taking on the role of clinical supervisor, as believing in your own abilities will help you become more competent and effective. You may wish to consider the following questions as you begin to take on the challenge of becoming a supervisor.

Reflective activity

- What experience of clinical supervision would you least expect from your own supervisor?
- What competences do you have to start supervising?
- What would your colleagues, past and present, say your strengths are in this role?
- What would they say are areas for you to develop?
- How can you acquire any more experience that you still feel you need?
- What initiatives can you put in place to remain competent?
- Do you feel that you are a genuine role model to your supervisee?

For several years now clinical supervision has been emerging in the healthcare professions, and various recommendations for its introduction and implementation in the workplace have been put forward (Kohner 1994). The means to deliver and implement clinical supervision in the workplace can, and will, be diverse. For example, arranging protected time for supervision sessions to take place in a busy ward environment will require a different system from that used by supervisors who work in the community and organize their own caseload. There are vast numbers of published articles and a number of books that examine, consider the recommendations and detail the implementation process, with all the issues, dynamics, agendas that will arise. For the healthcare professions, Bond and Holland (1998) do this comprehensively, as does Driscoll (2000). I do not wish to expand on this here as it will vary across organizations and you may not be involved in the process. However, it is important for you to acknowledge and have awareness of guidelines for the introduction of clinical supervision, as, after all, that is what you will be doing.

In 1994 the King's Fund Centre published a report that offers guidelines for the introduction of supervision (see box). These guidelines were derived from practice and are still relevant as a general framework. In particular, they highlight some of the issues that need to be discussed with managers and educators.

Guidelines for the introduction of clinical supervision

1 Before introducing clinical supervision, its purpose should be discussed and clearly defined. This definition should be informed by a theoretical understanding of the role and function of supervision and equally by a practical understanding of the circumstances and needs of the unit and its staff.
2 All staff should be involved in the process of planning and introducing a system of clinical supervision.
3 Careful consideration should be given to the qualifications, skills and experience required of supervisors, and to their ability to meet the individual needs of supervisees.
4 All supervisors should be given opportunities to receive training and learn the skills that are needed to provide supervision that is both constructive and supportive. Those who receive supervision should have similar opportunities to learn about their role as supervisees.
5 All supervisors should also receive supervision, in order to monitor and develop the quality of supervision they provide.
6 Supervision should be available to all practitioners, regardless of seniority.
7 The content of supervision should be carefully defined, with boundaries agreed about *what is* and *is not* to be dealt with in supervision time. The processes to be used should also be made clear.
8 The relationship between supervisor and supervisee should be formally constituted. Ground rules should be negotiated and agreed.
9 It is essential that clinical supervision is monitored and evaluated. Supervisees and supervisors should play an equal part in these procedures.
10 Individual units need the support of their employing authority to implement and maintain a system of clinical supervision.

Source: King's Fund Centre 1994

Relevant collaboration with others

From the above guidelines it is clear that there needs to be collaboration with other parties and that commitment and training are necessary. Motivation and dedication will be needed, but you will be unable to sustain these on your own and to stay effective without the ongoing support of relevant other parties. To continue with the theme of clinical supervision as a learning journey, you may want to ask yourself: Do I want to be secure in the middle of the boat or do I take up the challenges of holding on to the sides on my own? Beginning supervision often feels as though you are testing the waters and getting your feet wet and, of course, that is (figuratively speaking) what you have to do. It will, however, be helpful not only to have the support of other significant parties, but also to continually keep them on board, in view and involved with the supervision process. So, who are the relevant other parties? One way to conceptualize this can be seen in Figure 1.1.

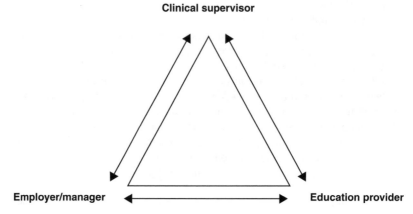

Clinical supervisor

Employer/manager   **Education provider**

FIGURE 1.1 Triangle for supervision implementation. (Adapted from Hughes and Pengelly 1997)

Figure 1.1 shows the desired situation between you the clinical supervisor, your employer or manager and your education provider. These should be the significant parties involved in collaboration to ensure the quality and effectiveness of the clinical supervision that has been, or is going to be, implemented. As Figure 1.1 indicates, there needs to be clear and open collaboration between the three parties. I have found that this triangle is helpful to conceptualize the roles and the dynamics of the main players in establishing clinical supervision in the healthcare setting.

Each significant party needs to see and be in contact with the others, and all need to be within equal reach. Working partnerships will need to be developed and maintained if supervision is to be ongoing. Ask yourself who are you going to turn to and ask for support and guidance when problems or issues arise.

If the implementation process has been thoroughly researched and explored, and the arrangements are in place, then you are ready to take your first steps in supervision. Implementation may be on a large scale, where many other disciplines have been involved and firm foundations are in place, or on a much smaller, individual scale. However, training and education should have been undertaken to develop the skills, principles and roles needed in supervision. Providing clinical supervision is a responsibility and should not take

place without sufficient and suitable training. I am highlighting
acknowledge the responsibilities that other parties have in yʊ
development as a supervisor. There is a need to monitor the process anu
systems needed for successful and sustained delivery.

It is generally agreed that good employers look after their staff. In the pressured environment of healthcare, all healthcare staff should have the right to
access clinical supervision, and the supervisor the right to be fully supported
by those around them. As a supervisor, you will have responsibility for maintaining the supervision process within the organizational system in addition
to the pressures of your workload. It is therefore vital that you have the full
backing of your employer and manager. As the supervision sessions will be
taking place during working hours, you will also need the support of colleagues to enable you to fulfil the role. To ensure, then, that your first steps
into clinical supervision are effective, it is envisaged that a protocol has been
formulated and agreed by the relevant parties. A suggested protocol for the
desired situation would be as follows:

- The introduction and implementation of clinical supervision has resulted
  from detailed preparation and negotiation.
- There are clear contracts and expectations on all sides.
- All role definitions are clear.
- The aims and objectives of clinical supervision are agreed.
- Adequate training is provided.
- There is provision for supervisors' own clinical supervision.

Training for clinical supervision

Often, supervisors have learnt their skills and techniques from their own
supervisors, and this is a valid and important way of learning. Former supervisors are often excellent and competent role models; however, the opposite
can also be true. The standards and practice of supervision being offered may
have been less than desirable in meeting the needs of the supervisee or the
organization. This may well influence how the new supervisor operates and
their understanding of the role. Clinical supervisors need to develop their own
style and not attempt to emulate the style of others. Learn from your own
experience alongside developing new knowledge, understandings and experiences that a competent training programme can offer.

What constitutes a competent training programme? At the time of writing
there are no clear guidelines or recommendations of a suitable length of course
or content. Inevitably, the length of programmes will be variable, but it should
be intended to suit the particular needs and context of the organization. The
content needs to be designed and delivered by the relevant parties who are

committed to clinical supervision and have collaborated to produce a competent programme. I list below some questions to raise with your service and education providers regarding the training that is or will be on offer:

- What is the length of the programme and how has that been determined? If it is minimal, for example less than four days, then ask how is that justified and whether there are to be further updates and workshops.
- What content does it cover?
- Will the training prepare me adequately to become a clinical supervisor, and how will this be assessed and monitored?
- Is the training and experience going to be largely experiential? (This would more realistically convey and suit the material to be offered.)
- Will there be plenty of opportunity to give and receive constructive feedback with other participants and the programme leaders?
- What training is being offered to the supervisee? For example, is there to be awareness-raising sessions on the purpose of supervision, reflective practice and training on how to use clinical supervision to full benefit.

While talking to other relevant parties, listen out for their enthusiasm, dedication and rationale towards clinical supervision. This may begin to tell you something about their overall commitment or whether they are merely doing this as part of their role requirement and job description.

Reflective activity

Focus and look back on the training programme you have undertaken and ask yourself:

- What did you value the most?
- What did you value the least?
- From the programme content, what would you have liked more of? Less of?
- Overall, did the programme fulfil its objectives? If not, why not?
- Would you at some point in the future contribute to a supervision training programme?

Conclusion

This chapter has introduced clinical supervision, focusing on important issues and understandings that a beginning supervisor needs to be aware of and have in place before commencement. The next chapter focuses on the first meeting and making a supervision contract.

Key learning points

- In being able to define clinical supervision you are also able to distinguish it from other, similar activities.
- It is important to understand the antecedents of clinical supervision as well as emerging factors that commend its implementation in practice.
- As a healthcare professional you will have many transferable skills to use in the role of supervisor. However, you need first to understand the specific aims and objectives of supervision.
- Understanding the main functions of clinical supervision will help keep you focused on its aims and objectives.
- As a new supervisor, you have understanding of the importance and value of collaboration with the significant other parties involved to provide you with support and training.

2

What to Cover at a First Meeting

Chapter outcomes

By reading this chapter, doing the reflective activities, and integrating the material into your supervision practice, you should be able to:

- Recognize the importance of a clinical supervision contract.
- Acknowledge the essential elements in a supervision contract.
- Develop negotiations regarding rights and responsibilities for the supervisor and supervisee.
- Become aware of effective contributions to the supervision relationship.
- Acknowledge some important points to discuss and consider at a first supervision meeting.
- Acknowledge the responsibilities and requirements regarding the practicalities of arranging supervision meetings.
- Understand the issues regarding taking notes, record keeping and related legal matters.
- Introduce a clinical supervision contract.

Introduction

Since the Kohner (1994) report on clinical supervision, almost all the policies and documents from various trusts and healthcare agencies advocate a contract to be agreed in the initial implementation stages for supervision (Power 1999). You will need to identify your own organization's prescribed contract of agreement for the supervisor and supervisee. It is important that you read this document. If you are going to be responsible for formulating the contract I strongly urge you to follow the guidelines in this chapter. That is also assuming that you have the support of your organization in implementing one-to-one supervision and that there are agreed expectations and responsibilities. I offer some examples of a contract at the end of this chapter.

The purpose of a supervision contract

As supervision has a specific purpose and there will be limited time for it to take place, it is generally agreed that this arrangement should have a contract. Brown and Bourne (1996) purport that a contract is a necessary starting point to any supervision relationship. You might find the term 'contract' off-putting at first for various reasons, or it may be new to you in the context of helping relationships. It may help to consider the contract as an agreement between the two of you, and you may wish to refer to it verbally as a 'working agreement' as you are both establishing the principles and practicalities of supervision together.

The supervision process is a formal agreement which differs from other support systems. What makes it different is the agreement to establish a working relationship for the objectives of supervision to be carried out. It is an interpersonal process of which the success will depend heavily upon the quality of the relationship between the supervisor and supervisee. This supportive relationship has been shown to be essential to effective supervision (Berger and Buchholz 1993; Simms 1993). A contract, therefore, will lay the foundation on which to build the supervision relationship. This not only makes the task in hand a joint responsibility, but also defines ways the relationship may best work to cultivate and nourish that task. Samuel Goldwyn (1879–1974) is quoted as saying that a verbal contract isn't worth the paper it is written on, but the general point is to make the contract a written one.

Reflective activity

- Make a list of what you consider to be the advantages of having a contract – either written or verbal – for clinical supervision.
- Would there be any disadvantages?

It may help to think of your own experiences of being in supervision, or similar situations and if having a clearer working agreement would have helped with any difficulties that emerged.

Essential elements of a supervision contract

The contract that is to be negotiated between the supervisor and the supervisee and documented in order to underpin the supervisory relationship should, first and foremost, include the following:

- The method of supervision being offered – one-to-one or group.
- Rights and responsibilities – ground rules for the nature of the relationship.
- Goals, aims and objectives for clinical supervision – agreed and specific.
- What to bring to supervision – agreed boundaries for content of sessions.
- Confidentiality – what action should be taken in relation to unsafe or unprofessional practice, and the limits of that action.

It should also set out details of:

- The frequency of the meeting.
- The time for each session and the duration of each session.
- The venue.
- Privacy.
- The method of recording and note taking.
- Storage of records.
- Provision for non-attendance, sickness, holiday etc., and how to cancel pre-arranged sessions.
- Evaluation of satisfaction with sessions.
- Review of the contract – how and when.

To summarize the above and for a quick checklist, remember the three Rs that are to be covered by the contract:

- **Roles**
- **Requirements**
- **Responsibilities**

Negotiation of rights and responsibilities

One of the most important elements of a supervision contract is the rights and responsibilities that you both undertake to agree on. You need to remember that supervision '*is always the practitioner's development space*' (Johns 2004: 81). Therefore, the supervisee has the right to be very much included in the negotiations and discussions that will constitute the working agreement and contract.

A supervision contract needs to outline the key responsibilities of the supervisor and supervisee as these are both individual and dual responsibilities. Read the rights and responsibilities of the clinical supervisor and of the supervisee, which have been adapted from Bond and Holland (1998) in the box below.

Rights and responsibilities

Rights of the supervisee in clinical supervision

- To have choice about the mode of supervision and choice of supervisor with due regard to any current constraints.
- To be treated with respect as an equal partner in the supervision relationship.
- To be involved in making any decisions that affect the agreements.
- To set the agenda to meet your own professional needs.
- To confidentiality, with the exception of revealing anything that breaks the law, trust policy or professional code of conduct.
- To protected time, e.g. minimum of one hour every month, for the clinical supervision to take place.
- To protected space, in private with no interruptions.
- To be able to talk about any difficulties and vulnerable feelings, if the supervisee so wishes, without being criticized for having those vulnerabilities.
- No record to be kept on personal issues that have been talked about.

Responsibilities of the supervisee in clinical supervision

- To attend a minimum of one hour every month and to provide evidence of this to your line manager.
- To assert yourself in negotiating who will be your clinical supervisor.
- To prepare for clinical supervision by identifying clinical/professional issues upon which you wish to reflect.
- To ask for particular help or other attention with the focus of reflecting on, developing and improving professional practice with the support of the supervisor.
- To time by giving the appointments a high priority and arriving punctually.
- To arrange cover so that you can attend clinical supervision.
- To make and follow through action plans that arise from your reflection.
- To be open to, or be prepared to, challenge by explaining or justifying actions in the context of constructive feedback, and not to interpret challenge as personal attacks or discriminatory practice.
- To give feedback to the supervisor about the facilitation, e.g. what is most helpful, what is least helpful.
- To use the time to reflect in depth on issues affecting clinical/professional practice and avoiding non-productive conversation.

- Where appropriate, to challenge any behaviour which is insulting or personally hurtful to you or others.

Rights of the clinical supervisor

- To be treated as an equal partner in the clinical supervision relationship, not blamed for any shortcomings of the supervisee or organization.
- To break confidentiality only in relation to the agreed contract.
- To refuse requests which make inappropriate demands on you in your role as supervisor, e.g. outside interference from the supervisee's colleagues or manager or inappropriate requests from the supervisee.
- To set personal and professional boundaries on what issues you listen to the supervisee talking about.
- To choose whether or not to work with a person as their clinical supervisor.
- To take steps to withdraw from the clinical supervision relationship if you have difficulties in meeting the commitment.

Responsibilities of the clinical supervisor

- To prepare for the supervision session, ensuring no interruptions, settling yourself beforehand and remembering previous sessions.
- To be reliable, sticking to appointments, time boundaries, supervision contract and agreed confidentiality.
- To ensure that management or educational assessment is not part of the role and to keep session time purely within the clinical supervision contract.
- To offer first aid counselling for current burning issues with the focus on maintaining quality professional practice in spite of personal difficulties.
- To encourage the supervisee to seek specialist help or advice when necessary.
- To challenge any behaviour that the supervisee displays or talks about which gives you concern about their practice, development or use of supervision.
- To ensure that you have the necessary back-up, e.g. your own supervision and support system.
- Where appropriate to challenge any behaviour which is insulting or personally hurtful to you or others.

Source: Adapted from Bond and Holland 1998

Reflective activity

- Do you feel that you have the necessary skills and resources to discuss what is being asked and suggested by the above rights and responsibilities?
- Do you feel you that have the necessary skills and resources to offer what is being asked for and suggested by the above rights and responsibilities?

- Which rights and responsibilities raise the most anxiety for you?
- Which may raise the most anxiety for your supervisee?
- Are there any other rights and responsibilities that you would add to these suggestions?

The rights and responsibilities listed above can be a very useful starting place for discussions and negotiations with your supervisee in making a contract. Such a list allows for the parameters and boundaries of the relationship to be made clear. While creating a working alliance together it will also serve to minimize and guard against the abuse of power (Hewson 1999).

Having reflected on and addressed the questions in the last activity you may be now more aware of, and prepared to address these, in the first session. You may want to have your own written copy available at the first meeting and to think about how you will introduce these. You may want to consider writing to your supervisee beforehand, briefly introducing yourself and stating that the intentions of your first meeting will be to discuss the workings of the supervision relationship. This can serve several purposes: to break the ice, to be a welcome note, and to set the tone of the sessions by indicating that they are for the supervisee's benefit and that the relationship is an equal and shared responsibility. Make this a golden opportunity to launch the beginnings of your working relationship together. Start as you mean to continue by establishing your style, so your supervisee begins to experience how you are to work with as a supervisor. If you make this process creative, supportive and challenging, with a focus on the aims and objectives, you set the scene for effective supervision. Thought and planning, as well as having the courage of your convictions, will be needed. Laying the foundations on rock rather than sand will have its rewards. The relationship needs to be strong and enduring, so put in the effort for the long haul, commit to the relationship. The more you put in the more you may reap (Covey 1992). This theme is continued in the next section and is well worth considering as you take your first steps into supervising.

Making contributions to the supervision relationship

Covey (1992) uses the metaphor of an 'emotional bank account' as a way of maintaining and improving relationships and says it is a way to describe *'the amount of trust that's been built up in a relationship'* (p. 188). I find this a very useful image that can be applied to elements of the supervision relationship. One way to think about the relationship you are embarking upon is to consider it as being like opening a bank account. The context here is to think of it as an emotional bank account, one that you can make deposits into and, just like a real bank account, make withdrawals from. The emotional units that

Covey speaks of are centred on trust, which is an essential quality of the relationship. You may also view it as an expression of your credibility with your supervisee, with the more you deposit into the account, the healthier the balance, or, in real terms, the relationship, will be. However, because we are human and not perfect, things can interfere with our lives and distract us from putting all we might into a supervision relationship. Therefore, withdrawals will occur. Withdrawals happen when your actions hurt a person or impair the relationship in some way. Although these types of withdrawals will not have been intentional, often we are busy and other things do get in the way. What you need to be aware of is the effect it can have on the other person: they may well feel let down and be asking themself 'are these sessions really going to benefit me?' It will be wise to consider throughout the relationship the commitment you are putting in and the value you are placing on it. In the box below is a list of deposits that you can put into the relationship and the possible withdrawals that might take place.

Build up your account deposits from the beginning

- A warm welcome and small act of kindness can go a long way.
- Display your enthusiasm for clinical supervision and for your supervisee.
- Fully engage your supervisee in the contract process as an equal partner.
- Get to know and take interest in your supervisee as a person and unique human being. Ask yourself, for example, what makes them tick? What are their strengths? What are their qualities?
- Always end the meetings by giving positive feedback to the supervisee.

Some likely withdrawals

- Being late and keeping your supervisee waiting.
- Appearing to be in a hurry during the session.
- Having so many other things on your mind that you find it difficult to fully engage and concentrate.
- Just having a very bad day.
- Using the session to offload and talk about your own stress and work-related issues.

The above list of deposits shows just some ways you can begin to build and establish the relationship from the opening session. You may already have put forward a welcoming gesture by sending out some information beforehand. You will have every opportunity as the trust and relationship grows to use your skills and techniques to develop the supervision process and experience.

Withdrawals that can happen are due to a lack of skill or to inexperience or misjudgement in self-awareness and insight. When you sense that the relationship with your supervisee is stuck or going downhill, think about whether any withdrawals may have occurred recently and whether you have been taking out more than you have been putting in. Ask yourself some of the following questions:

- Am I making honest, genuine and positive 'deposits'?
- In what criteria am I 'overdrawn'?
- How will I address this?

Becoming quickly aware of any withdrawals you make is a first step to re-addressing the positive balance of the supervision relationship. There may be many external obstacles hindering your ability to provide effective supervision. These can have the effect of making a withdrawal from your supervision account. So make sure you have certain deposits in place for you, such as the following.

- Provision for your own supervision.
- Support from managers and colleagues.
- A suitable and accessible venue.
- Access to training and other support systems for clinical supervisors.

Putting in a little extra

Good self-awareness will enable you generally to keep a focus on and maintain the balance of a healthy supervision relationship. It is impossible to be the greatest supervisor ever, yet you can do small things which often have a great effect:

- **Keep commitments**. Keeping commitments by following up any requests made to you and any promises you make during sessions are major deposits. The breaking of these can make for withdrawals.
- **Small acts of human kindness**. Small courtesies and compliments are important deposits. Acts of disrespect make for large withdrawals. Maintaining positive energy by allowing a spirit of goodwill and kindness to permeate the supervision relationship I consider to be not only a first step but a continuing step to take. Eliminating blame, criticism, judgements, pettiness and other negative characteristics in our lives in general are terrific acts of kindness.
- **Understand your supervisee**. Really get to know your supervisee over the period of time you spend with them. Knowing and understanding them both as a healthcare worker and as a person are most important deposits. After getting to know your supervisee you will be able to give personalized

feedback. For example, 'You have a real strength in promoting your ideas and backing them up with evidence. You have demonstrated that with me and in your workplace.'

- **Get to know them as a person**. You have a little time before the session gets under way and again once the session has completed. Take this opportunity to talk about small details that your supervisee has mentioned about family or other personal interests. For example, 'When is your next weekend away walking? I imagine you find that a good way to get away from the pressures of work.' Or, 'How is the saxophone practice going? You mentioned you started lessons.' As well as demonstrating your interest it communicates that you think about them as a person.

- **Apologize for small mistakes**. Own up and do not make excuses. This will demonstrate your humanness, genuineness, sincerity and honesty. For example, 'I was wrong to interrupt like that. I really should have given you more time to think.' Or, 'Sorry, I must not have been fully paying attention to you last time; I had forgotten that that had happened.'

Getting started with the first meeting

Once you have your first meeting organized, you will no doubt be asking yourself, 'how do I start and what may be asked of me?' The following suggested starting points may provide some answers.

- Share some details about your careers and experience, past and present.
- Mention briefly the circumstances that have brought you both here.
- Discuss the expectations and aims of clinical supervision.
- Discuss previous experience of clinical supervision.
- Discuss any anxieties about the process.

However you choose to start the first meeting, think about how you are going to introduce yourself. Remember that you only have one chance to make a good first impression. Also remember the importance of body language and that spoken words are only a fraction of the messages we send (Argyle 1975).

If, like me, you have worked in the helping professions for many years, it has probably been many years since your initial training in communication skills. When we are constantly in a role and communicating from a position of expertise or authority we can let our good habits slip and become complacent with regard to communicating our interest and listening to others. When did you last receive constructive feedback on your presentation and inter- and intrapersonal skills, for example?

We want to give a good impression of the task and role for which the supervisee has chosen us. So greet with gestures of enthusiasm. Following on from the initial welcome, the supervisee is probably expecting you to ask some questions about them. It will help to take charge of the session at this point and to seek to create an atmosphere that is relaxed, non-threatening and enquiring. Use their name, having earlier established how they like to be addressed, and ask an open question such as, 'What would you like to tell me about your current area of work and the role you have?'

This gives the supervisee a certain amount of freedom and opportunity to share with you what they see as relevant. You can then fill in some gaps with more specific questions such as asking about previous clinical experience. Be careful at this stage not to pepper the supervisee with too many questions; remember this is their time and space. Asking too many questions at the start of something new often betrays something of our own anxiety about starting the actual supervision, so we play safe and do something that we know how to do and keeps us in control.

Sharing some information about your background and work experience allows the supervisee to get to know you. Be careful, though, not to overload them or to take this as an opportunity to talk about yourself. Share, for now, what you feel is relevant to the supervisee. You may want to do this by asking the supervisee what they want to know about you. This can signal that from the beginning of the relationship there is to be an equal balance. You will want to establish a balanced relationship in many aspects of the process and you can start here by inviting and encouraging the supervisee to ask questions. From the very beginning this can stimulate and develop the inquisitiveness of the supervisee. This can also help foster the position that they are taking responsibility for the main agenda for the sessions, within the context and objectives of clinical supervision.

What has brought us here? Expectations for supervision

It is important to ask your supervisee about the circumstances which have brought them to you and the nature of their supervision experience. By raising these subjects you are inviting the supervisee to express their thoughts about why they are choosing to come to supervision at this present time. This could be for a variety of reasons which may have a bearing on how the first few sessions will take effect.

The issue of the supervisee's right to choose their supervisor is pertinent here. In the ideal situation they should have that right, but this is always going to be limited to some degree by a multitude of resource and organizational issues. However, negotiation, and perhaps compromise, will need to take place regarding the choice of supervisor (Johns 2004). It is highly desirable that the supervisee has been able to choose you as their supervisor and they are fully willing to take part.

Trust is an integral component of clinical supervision, so the supervisee in the ideal scenario would have identified a professional whom they feel able to trust and to benefit from professionally. Circumstances may not have permitted free choice and they were allocated to you. If this is the case then explore how they feel about working with you and any anxieties that they might have. It may, of course, be difficult for the supervisee to disclose these things, especially when put on the spot. You therefore may want to use the skill of empathic reflecting and say something to the effect of, 'I'm aware you have been allocated to me rather than your having more free choice. I'm wondering if that raises any anxieties for you, perhaps on the issue of trust?' This question indicates that you have been thinking about the situation and how they might be feeling. From this first step into supervision you are creating a climate of openness and honesty that is vital to the development of the relationship. It also demonstrates that you are taking a risk by raising the issue for the benefit of the task in hand.

When you start out, ask your supervisee if they have had any previous experience of supervision. This gives them an opportunity to talk about any negatives as well as the positives. You may use this as an evaluation in considering what was good and not so good about the experience. If they have had a negative experiences, ask, 'What are some ways that we could work together to avoid that happening?', or, 'What could I do differently to make this more positive for you?' Avoid, however, going into any personal detail about a previous supervisor; keep it focused on the supervision that is to take place between you both in the here and now. This can be an opening to raise any issues for your working relationship and how these may be addressed. You are creating here a mutual relationship which is open to negotiation.

Those questions offer the opportunity to talk about any anxieties they may have about taking up supervision and how those might be reduced. Go back and look over the rights and responsibilities that were listed earlier in this chapter: both of you can consider what you would want to include in your contract and how this experience can be more positive.

If the supervisee has had a positive experience, validate it and then ask, 'What would you like from me to maintain that?' and, 'How might we make this experience of supervision even more beneficial for you?'

If, however, this is a new experience for your supervisee, ask similar questions in the nature of, 'What are your hopes and expectations for these sessions?', and, 'What are some of your worst fears?' These are ways to balance out the preconceived ideas the supervisee may have.

Take mental notes to the responses that are offered. Write these down for your own personal notes as soon as possible after the session has finished, or you may prefer to do this as you go along during the session – but be sure to be open with them what you are noting down and the reasons for this.

Questions that the supervisee may ask you

Questions you may be asked include:
- How long have you been a supervisor?
- What training have you had to be a supervisor?
- What is expected of me in supervision?
- How are these sessions going to work?

Reflective activity

- What other questions might be asked of you at a first meeting?
- What questions did you ask at your first supervision session?
- What questions did you not ask but wish you had?

Think about what you are to tell your supervisee of your experience of supervision. You may already have made a supervision CV and profile that was mentioned in Chapter 1. It will help to remind yourself of the aims and purposes of clinical supervision and to have a definition that you have formulated from the background information and training in supervision that you have experienced. This can be an opening to demonstrate your own commitment, motivation and enthusiasm, by self-disclosing how you have used, and do use, clinical supervision, and the benefits it has. This is also a chance to raise awareness of the real purpose of clinical supervision.

I subscribe to the view of Faugier (1996), who stated that if supervision is not about improving patient care then there is no real need for it. Take this opening exchange as another golden opportunity to emphasize that clinical supervision is about improving patient care and well-being. Give some brief examples from your own experience to that effect. By explaining how you have used the supervision experience, you can go some way towards helping the supervisee to understand what is to be expected of them and how the sessions are to work. Offer a succinct example of when supervision really benefited you. This can demonstrate how it can work, and, by self-disclosing, you are taking a risk that can lay the foundations for your supervisee to take risks in future sessions.

This may be your first supervision session as a supervisor and it will be both genuine and honest to state that fact, if it is to serve a purpose for the supervisee. For example, you may say something like: 'Part of me is feeling rather anxious, as perhaps you are. This also is my first time in this role, but I have been looking forward very much to working and learning with you.' If said in a manner that expresses both warmth and confidence to the supervisee, such a statement conveys how you feel, and has the intention of being empathic and communicates enthusiasm.

Contracting for supervision: agreeing the practicalities

There are a number of practicalities that need arranging when you begin to provide supervision. These are outlined below.

Location

The location where supervision is to take place should be jointly agreed and as convenient as possible for both parties to get to. The environment should also be as free as possible from distractions and interruptions. As the supervisor, you will need to consider the most suitable location as regards the needs of your supervisee. Will it be more beneficial to create a reflective and learning climate for the venue to be in a neutral location rather than the work area? This may not be possible for a variety of reasons but is something you will both need to negotiate.

Frequency

You will both need to decide how often the supervision sessions should take place. As the supervisor, you will need to assess a workable frequency bearing in mind the functions and purpose of supervision and taking into account any other forms of support your supervisee is receiving. A general rule for individual supervision would be once a month. Any longer than this begs the question, is it really fulfilling the objectives and intentions of clinical supervision? The objectives of supervision are threefold: a regular means of developing quality and safe practice, an opportunity to learn and reflect on practice, and a place to receive support for feelings and emotions that arise from practice. I believe that one hour once a month is the minimum amount of time needed to carry out these objectives. Once the frequency of the sessions has been determined, then negotiate how long the session will last. I would suggest one hour as that tends to be a maximum amount of time for your concentrated listening and attention span. This so-called fifty minute hour allows for a few minutes at the start to get settled in and a few minutes at the end for clarification of the next meeting and saying goodbye. I have always found it beneficial to try to keep to the same day and time per month. Not only does this help to keep it in your memory, but you can also then make it an established commitment in your diary and others will also become aware of this priority as well. You will also need to agree a method by which the sessions may be cancelled. Holidays, illness and exceptional circumstances would be legitimate reasons. Cancellations should be pre-arranged or, whenever possible, at least 24 hours' notice given. You may agree that it is the responsibility of the person who cancels to rearrange the next session.

Note taking and record keeping

The taking of notes and record keeping for clinical supervision is a rather contentious and sensitive issue, and the legal aspects are not absolute.

Diamond (1998a, b) was among the first authors to highlight this issue, and it would appear that clinical supervision records could, might or may find themselves in a court of law if disciplinary procedures were to be taken against either the supervisee or the supervisor. Cutcliffe (2000) refers to the potential minefield of legal, accountability and ethical issues and add that this may cause some to be hesitant of taking up the role of supervisor. Thankfully, I do not feel this has been the case. There does need to be more clarity regarding the legal aspects and related issues in clinical supervision, but I will leave that investigation in the hands of those more experienced in such matters. I will, however, discuss legal issues next and will attempt to keep it simple.

Legal issues

Diamond (1998a) states the where clinical supervision is a requirement of the employment contract and the employer resources the provision, the employer owns any records and has a right to access records of attendance. If disciplinary proceedings were to take place that involve either supervisor or the supervisee, and and their supervision is relevant to the issue arising, then the employer would have the right to access records. Diamond also states the law courts are in a position to subpoena records. I would want to agree with Bond and Holland (1998) who state that this would be very unlikely. I share the view of Cutcliffe (2000) and Driscoll (2007), among other authors, who advocate that these legal issues should not deter any persons from being involved in supervision or from becoming a supervisor. In fact I believe that an awareness of the legal requirements and responsibilities helps the supervisor to set a professional standard that will be both reliable with respect to keeping records of attendance and functional with respect to the taking of notes. A fundamental aim of supervision is to enable and support best practice with your supervisee, so it would be logical to demonstrate best practice in record keeping.

It would appear to be the case that where supervision is a more voluntary arrangement and not resourced by your employer, and where it takes place outside of your employer's time, then records are owned by the supervisor. The most desirable arrangement, however, is for supervision to be conducted with the full backing of your employer. Whatever the position, confidentiality must be addressed and records documented in such a way that safe practice – not just safe supervisory practice – is demonstrated. Records need not be viewed in a suspicious or negative way. On the contrary, they can demonstrate that both parties are engaging in a supervisory process that is professional, safe and effective.

Guidelines for record keeping

The following can be determined and agreed by you both by asking what will be the most beneficial way:

- To keep the balance of power equal in the supervision relationship. This can be achieved by always agreeing and sharing any recorded notes with the supervisee.
- To establish where the records are to be kept, by whom, and who else may have access to them.

All written records should include:

- Time and date, name of supervisor and supervisee.
- A general outline of the issues raised and discussed and any outcomes or actions following supervision.
- Any general themes of session content which have been decided upon and which can be used for evaluation purposes. These could be grouped under the headings of:
  - Normative: when discussions have centred on direct client care: case reviews and time management, for example.
  - Formative: when discussions have centred on personal and professional development issues and learning outcomes, for example.
  - Restorative: when discussions have centred on general offloading of feelings and frustrations, or and on stress management, for example.

However, keep in mind the following guidelines.

- Keep a note of topics and issues discussed using just key words or headings.
- Avoid any specific personal information that could identify individuals.
- For supervisees who have ongoing caseloads you may need to establish how you are to identify cases that need regular monitoring. The use of an initial or code could be used to aid your memory.

Reflective activity

When taking your first steps and becoming a supervisor ask yourself the following questions regarding record keeping:

- What is the policy or expectation of my organization on keeping notes and records?
- How can I / we make best use of any records for audit purposes and evaluating the effectiveness of clinical supervision?
- Who owns the notes and records?
- Who has access to them?
- Where am I to keep them and for how long?

A simple example of a form for keeping supervision records is offered in Figure 2.1. I have left the boxes open to allow you to formulate your own criteria bearing in mind the guidelines for record keeping.

RECORD OF SUPERVISION	Supervisor...
Agenda/topics brought to supervision	Supervision..
Discussion notes	Action/outcomes

Signed ....Supervisee   Signed ....Supervisor

Date ....

DATE OF NEXT MEETING.................................

FIGURE 2.1 Example sheet for recording clinical supervision content

Introducing and making a contract

When you first start work with your supervisee, make clear the reasons for a contract by giving information of what you are doing and why. The following are some examples you could use when introducing a supervision contract:

- 'I would like us to look at some rights and responsibilities that have been suggested for us both to aware of for supervision to take place. These sessions are for you, and I feel it will be valuable for me to have your views, and I will answer any questions you may have.'
- 'I am asking you to consider these aspects of the contract because it is important that you can get the most out of this agreement we are making together.'
- 'It is important that you tell me what you need as we go along as it will give me some idea of how I could best enable that.'
- 'I would like to ask you if you feel there is anything I have missed.'
- 'It is important that, having looked at these together, we have shared understanding. Perhaps we should summarize the main points of our contract?'

McLeod (2007) advocates that it is valuable to consider the use of pronouns in counselling conversations, and in particular the use of the words 'I' and 'we'. I feel the usage transfers equally here to conversations in supervision and can help to make the relationship more intimate and collaborative. In addition, the use of summarizing, if introduced early in the relationship, can foster a feeling of future progress, one of anticipation that this is to be a joint working relationship. It can also have the effect of reassurance: the supervisee knows that you have understood and that this is a shared responsibility with mutual aims.

You may prefer to use the phrase 'working agreement' when referring to the contract as this sounds rather more friendly and implies a joint responsibility. Two examples of a supervision contract are offered below.

Example of a clinical supervision contract

1. The content of the Clinical Supervision session will be to:
- Review clinical practice.
- Discuss current problems / concerns.
- Discuss issues related to professional development.

The normative, formative and restorative functions of clinical supervision will be used as a conceptual framework.

2. The Clinical Supervision session will be held every ....for approximately ....hour(s).

---

3. Confidentiality between both supervisor and supervisee(s) will be strictly maintained in order that it will not be breached outside of the session unless otherwise agreed by both parties.

Confidentiality clause: All issues discussed will be in confidence, unless there is anything disclosed that affects the well-being of the supervisee or is detrimental to patients, professional practice, the team or the organization.

In the event of disclosure of information that constitutes malpractice or places the patient or organization at risk, action will be taken to inform the relevant line manager.

4. A record of attendance will be kept and may be provided for monitoring and audit. Written records of supervisory sessions may be recorded by the supervisor and agreed by the supervisee. Confidentiality and privacy will be maintained in accordance with the professional code of conduct. Both parties may also use a personal reflective journal.

5. We both agree that regular supervision is a commitment and should be cancelled only in the event of illness or crisis. Notice will be given and it is the responsibility of the person who cancels to rearrange the session.

6. Both parties will participate in formal evaluation of supervisory meetings after .... months. Evaluation feedback will be used constructively and may be disclosed to other parties.

7. In the event of the supervisory partnership being ineffective or any difficulties arising, either party can choose to terminate the contract after full discussion and agreement by both parties.

8. In the event of termination of a supervision contract it is the supervisee's responsibility to approach and agree an alternative supervisor and supervision contract.

9. We agree to abide by the terms set out in this Clinical Supervision contract.

Name ....

Signature ....(Supervisee) Date ....

Name ....

Signature ....(Supervisor) Date ....

The above contract clearly outlines the functions of supervision and could be possibly be adapted for use in most supervision agreements. You could add specific ground rules to suit the context.

Another example of a supervision contract

We each agree:

- To meet at regular prearranged intervals for one hour.
- We will prioritize the sessions and inform each other as soon as possible if attendance is not possible and rearrange a following meeting.
- We will meet for six sessions and then review.
- The focus will be on any aspect of the supervisee's work.
- We will both abide by the Clinical Supervision policy of the organization by which we are employed.

My role as supervisee is to:

- Uphold ethical guidelines and professional standards with the aim to ensure and improve quality practice.
- Build a working relationship with you.
- Attend punctually supervision sessions that we organize.
- Help you to identify my work goals and agenda for supervision.
- Be open to feedback, change and consideration of alternative/improved methods of practice.
- Endeavour to complete tasks that we have agreed upon each session.
- Help me build my confidence, capabilities and skills in my work role.
- Express my thoughts and feelings about supervision and to give feedback to you.

I have read and agree to the organization's aims, objectives and policy on clinical supervision, which includes the guidelines on confidentiality and record keeping. I am familiar with its general operation.

This contract can be reviewed at any time upon my request to you and it will be reviewed annually.

Name .... Signature .... Date ....

My role as supervisor is to:

- Oversee the practice you do.
- Build a working relationship with you.
- Attend punctually supervision sessions that we organize.
- Help you to identify work goals and the agenda that you bring to supervision.
- Offer appropriate challenge and give constructive feedback to help you improve practice.
- Assist you to acquire knowledge and skills to use in your practice.
- Support you in your personal and professional development.

I have given you the organization's aims, objectives and policy on clinical supervision, which includes the guidelines on confidentiality and record keeping. I have read and agree to the organization's policy on clinical supervision and I am familiar with its general operation.

This contract can be reviewed at any time upon my request and it will be reviewed annually.

Name .... Signature .... Date ....

The above contract is offered as an alternative. It covers the same criteria but is perhaps more user friendly and less formal that the first one offered. Have a look and consider them both to see which would be more suited to your personal style and organization.

Reflective activity

If you are making your own contract:

- Does it include all the essential criteria?
- What else do you need to add?
- Has it been approved by all the other relevant parties?

If you are working with a contract that has been formulated by your organization/department:

- Are you satisfied with the content and able to work with it?
- Are there any pitfalls that you would want amended?
- What if problems arise with the contract? How will these be resolved?

Further questions for the supervisor to keep in mind:

- How will we know if the sessions are effective?
- Who have I identified to support me if any difficulties arise with the responsibilities I am taking on?

Conclusion

This chapter has focused on the significance of a clinical supervision contract and some of the main themes and issues to cover at a first meeting. The next chapter considers the value, importance and qualities that are needed to establish and maintain a clinical supervision relationship.

Key learning points

- It is important to understand the value of a collaborative written contract in enabling the requirements of clinical supervision to be met.
- Understanding the rights and responsibilities of both the supervisor and the supervisee will be a good starting point in establishing a supervision contract.
- As a supervisor, you will need knowledge of the supervision process, negotiation skills and commitment in establishing a contract with your supervisee.
- As a supervisor, you need to invest in the supervision relationship from the beginning: your enthusiasm and professionalism towards the task in hand can lay the foundation for a prosperous and efficient relationship.
- As a supervisor, you will know the essential criteria that need to be covered at a first meeting while keeping your supervisee engaged in the process and forming a collaborative relationship.
- Knowledge of the legal issues and your responsibilities regarding the keeping of notes and records will enable you to establish and maintain a professional approach, to the benefit of all concerned.

3

Qualities for a Healthy Supervision Relationship

Chapter outcomes

By reading this chapter, doing the reflective activities, and integrating the material into your supervision practice, you should be able to:

- Recognize qualities and characteristics for building an effective clinical supervision relationship.
- Begin to understand a key principle of person-centred theory.
- Acknowledge and develop the core conditions for a healthy supervision relationship.
- Understand the relevance of developing and sustaining self-awareness.
- Describe a framework for self-awareness.
- Possess some skills and techniques for giving constructive feedback.

Introduction

Among the many sentiments expressed by Carl Rogers when theorizing about human potential and development, was that healthy relationships create healthy people (Rogers 1980). To help bring out the potential, and therefore the best, in your supervisee, the relationship needs to be a prosperous one.

The foundation for that will be to create, establish and maintain a healthy relationship.

Reflective activity

Take a moment to think about Rogers's statement and of some of your own healthy relationships.

- What are the main characteristics of those relationships?
- What do you value most in them?
- What do you both contribute to them?

I would assume that you generally feel good about yourself and the other person in a healthy relationship. Make a note of your answers to the above activity so that you can begin to integrate those concepts into what you would consider to be appropriate in developing a supervision relationship. I, for example, would certainly consider that a healthy relationship is an honest and trusting one. I would also imagine that the many other attributes that you recognize in healthy relationships will be mentioned in this chapter, although perhaps not using the words you have used.

The essence of a supervision relationship

To develop a relationship that is to prosper and thrive, you, as supervisor, need to be honest and genuine in first creating that healthy relationship. Have a genuine desire to be a supervisor and for the task in hand, and view the relationship as a partnership or companionship, rather than as having expert and recipient roles.

I would like to suggest that you read the following credo by Thomas Gordon (1977) as I feel it is perfectly pertinent for a supervision relationship and the roles of both supervisor and supervisee. Dr Gordon wrote this credo as a basic philosophy for effective parent–child relationships. He then incorporated this belief in his training programmes on styles of leadership and effective human relationships. It offers a great deal of meaning as it represents what I feel we are striving for in a supervision relationship. After all, what's so funny about love, peace and understanding?

A credo for my relationships

You and I are in a relationship which I value and want to keep. Yet each of us is a separate person with unique needs and the right to meet those needs.

When you are having problems meeting your needs, I will try to listen with genuine acceptance, in order to facilitate your finding your own solutions instead of depending on mine. I also will try to respect your right to choose your own beliefs and develop your own values, different though they may be from mine.

However, when your behavior interferes with what I must do to get my own needs met, I will tell you openly and honestly how your behavior affects me, trusting that you respect my needs and feelings enough to try to change the behavior that is unacceptable to me. Also, whenever some behavior of mine is unacceptable to you, I hope you will tell me openly and honestly so I can try to change my behavior.

At those times when one of us cannot change to meet the other's needs, let us acknowledge that we have a conflict and commit ourselves to resolve each such conflict without either of us resorting to the use of power or authority to win at the expense of the other's losing. I respect your needs, but I also must respect my own. So let us always strive to search for a solution that will be acceptable to both of us. Your needs will be met, and so will mine – neither will lose, both will win.

In this way, you can continue to develop as a person through satisfying your needs, and so can I. Thus, ours can be a healthy relationship in which both of us can strive to become what we are capable of being. And we can continue to relate to each other with mutual respect, love, and peace.

Source: Gordon 1977: 261

Characteristics of a supervision relationship

If you are to view a supervision relationship as a partnership then you will need to make a connection with your supervisee. Nelson-Jones (2008: 28) argues that '*Connection is the essential characteristic of any relationship*'. In my experience, a successful clinical supervision relationship is created through a process of connecting with the other person. This needs to be a reliable connection that is built on nurturance, empathy and validation. This also needs to be a joined experience, and if it is to be sustained over time then the levels of connection will need to deepen. The relationship therefore needs to be both active and creative. Nicholls (2007) purports that these are essential elements for the partnership to flourish. I certainly agree that these are requisites for effective clinical supervision.

Faugier (1992) put forward a growth and support model that outlined effective characteristics for supervisors as facilitators. Her proposals follow a humanistic path and focus on the role of the supervisor as a provider of the essential ingredients for growth and support, thus allowing the supervisee to progress in the pursuit of clinical excellence. Faugier's (1992) model is well worth citing here as it also focuses on many of the qualities and characteristics that will help keep the relationship healthy.

One of the first steps for the supervisor is to create the essential characteristics for a healthy working relationship. I will also follow a humanistic path by considering how person-centred theory and the core conditions of helping can contribute to the development of connectedness and help the relationship to prosper.

Person-centred theory

Carl Rogers (1902–1987) is regarded as the spokesperson for humanistic psychology and is the originator of the person-centred approach. Through the discourse of his own studies he had become disillusioned with the behavioural and psychodynamic approaches in clinical psychology that were prevailing at that time. Rogers opposed those views that the therapist is the expert who was able to offer diagnosis and treatment in aspects of human growth, development and therapeutic change. His interest was how a person made meaning of their experiences, as he believed that people have the capacity and ability to identify, explore and ultimately resolve their own problems.

Person-centered theory holds a rather simplistic view of human nature. A key principle is that mentally healthy individuals are capable and have a tendency for self-direction in developing in a constructive and positive way. Another leading psychologist of the humanistic school was Abraham Maslow (1908–1970). It was from Maslow's concept of the 'hierarchy of human needs' (Maslow 1987) that Rogers developed the key themes and principles of his theory of what motivates the individual's growth and self-direction in reaching more of their own potential. Person-centred theory takes an optimistic view that human beings are rational, good, have unlimited potential and are capable both of assuming responsibility for themselves and of making choices. The key, however, when engaged in aspects of enabling this process in others, is the attitude of the helper and the quality of the therapeutic relationship. It is generally accepted that the principles of person-centred theory are essential in underpinning all types of helping relationships. They become therefore essential in establishing a clinical supervision relationship. These qualities are generally referred to as the core conditions. So, what are the characteristics and essential ingredients of the helping relationship that are fundamental to and underpin person-centred theory? The next section addresses this question.

The core conditions of helping and the supervision relationship

The following terms are commonly used to describe the core conditions, although some interpretations and a multitude of writings on the subject have used slightly different phrases. Egan (2002), for example, uses the term 'respect' when talking about unconditional positive regard. Genuineness is often linked with congruence. The quality of warmth is often used to convey a feeling, principally through non-verbal behaviour, that there is an active interest and a positive regard for the person. The core conditions are, then:

- Empathy
- Genuineness (or congruence)
- Acceptance (or warmth)
- Unconditional positive regard (or respect)

McCabe and Timmins (2006) and Hewitt et al. (2009) are among many authors in nursing that discuss and highlight the importance and value of the core conditions for helping relationships. They become therefore an obvious choice for the supervisor. Think of the relationship, which provides the core conditions, as the vehicle for therapeutic development and change.

These core conditions, or qualities, of helping relationships are grounded in the principles of the person-centred approach and humanistic theories of development. This theory of human development is also fundamental to teaching and learning (Gopee 2008). As a supervisor, you are also a facilitator of learning when functioning in the formative aspect of the role. Rogers (1983) views the teacher as a facilitator of learning, nurturing and providing resources while sharing their feelings and knowledge to the benefit of the other. Gopee (2008: 64) shares Rogers's philosophy and states: 'The prerequisites for being an effective facilitator of learning are awareness of self and being oneself in the teaching situation.' These prerequisites must be incorporated into the helper's way of being as a person, rather than just a set of tools or skills that can be accumulated. This calls for self-awareness in the supervisor in evaluating how effectively they are relating to the supervisee, interacting more consciously and with honest intent. Self-awareness is looked at in more detail later in the chapter. It is important first to consider the core conditions and to acknowledge the contribution they make to the supervision relationship.

Empathy (or empathic understanding)

Empathy means that you are able to see a situation or perspective from the other person's point of view. Empathy is different from sympathy. Sympathy implies that we feel for the other person; this can be in such close harmony that it affects us emotionally. In helping it can lead to over-identification and feeling sad or sorry for the other person unless we are able to contain our own feelings. We may not be able to deny our feelings of sympathy, and we should not try to do so, otherwise we might find it difficult to empathize with the person (Stein-Parbury 1993).

Empathy means that we are feeling with the other person and are able to grasp and participate in the other's thoughts and feelings without taking them fully within ourselves. It may be easier to acquire and thus demonstrate empathy if we have had a similar experience. The danger here is that our own feelings of that experience re-emerge in a negative or unresolved way. The supervisor needs to attempt to accurately see and understand the thoughts, feelings and meanings from the supervisee's perspective. We may not agree with the other's point of view but we can still have empathic understanding. Rogers (1961) adds most importantly that empathy is the ability to sense the other person's world as if it were your own, without losing the 'as if' quality. He places an emphasis on being sensitive in understanding the individual's feelings by not contaminating or confusing them with your own. We can be so full of our own opinions that we may not have the space for those of our supervisee. Empathy has been described as walking in someone else's shoes, experiencing not only how they may fit but also how they may pinch. It will help substantially if we first take off our own. The skill then is to communicate your empathic understanding to the supervisee in such a way that they feel fully heard, understood and accepted. There are limitations to being empathic, as unique individuals we all have different experiences of life, so we are unable to empathize truly with another person. However, through really listening and suspending judgement we can strive to see things more clearly from another's viewpoint.

Empathy brings the relationship closer together, and to be able to express and communicate empathy is an essential skill in developing understanding of the supervisee. As with any skill, we need to practise. It may help to think about progress rather than perfection. Practise with people you have a good relationship with by exploring their situation: check your empathy by stating in your own words what you understand of how they are thinking or feeling. Think of it as imagining aloud to them how it might be to be in their situation. You need, however, to really and fully listen from the 'as if' perspective and not your own. You also need to listen carefully and caringly. A task in supervision is to demonstrate understanding, of the supervisee's experience and understandings as they are revealed in the sessions, by empathic responding.

Some plausible supervisee statements about empathy

- 'She really understands how I feel.'
- 'She seems to know me from the inside.'
- 'There are certain moments when she puts my feelings into words.'
- 'She can read me like a book.'

A supervisee who experiences the supervisor's empathy and understanding is more likely to develop an increased self-empathy and self-acceptance which can be potent attributes for learning. Supervisees will also learn to trust you more, by your empathic responses in understanding how they view themselves, their work and what they care about.

Genuineness (or congruence)

Genuineness means that you are authentic and real in the relationship and role. The supervisee does not have to speculate what you are really like as a person, you are not screened by a professional facade, acting as the expert or playing the role. You are in the role of supervisor but you are being yourself. What you say should not conflict with how you feel. Own up to your mistakes, defects and shortcomings in the relationship when appropriate to do so. This may go against the training we have had as professional helpers, where we are advised to keep a professional distance. This behaviour may be appropriate in other roles you have but not in a supervision relationship. To be in touch with and acknowledge your significant thoughts and feelings within the relationship requires self-awareness. I use the words 'significant' and 'self-awareness' here because you are using your self-awareness to identify those of your personal thoughts that may be of benefit to the supervisee, and in doing so you are nurturing and developing the ongoing relationship. That is the factor which makes them significant. The term 'congruence' (Rogers 1961) refers to the fact that what the helper is thinking and feeling is consistent with what they are saying in the relationship. I like an interpretation of congruence used by Frankland and Sanders (1995), who use the word 'harmony'. In the context of supervision, this can be used to portray a harmonious attitude, for example:

- If you say you are interested and will help them explore a problem, your words should be consistent with your feelings.
- If you say 'good to see you again, how are you?', is this how you really feel? Is this reflected in body language and quality of voice?
- You do not avoid anything that is going to be important for the relationship.
- If you are clear yourself about the values and beliefs of supervision, you will more likely be able to express these in the relationship with the supervisee.
- You practise what you preach.
- Values and beliefs towards clinical supervision are evident in the relationship.
- Behaviour, such as interventions and actions, are consistent with attitudes about supervision.

- Genuineness encourages supervisee self-disclosure; appropriate supervisor disclosure enhances genuineness.
- Lack of congruence can cause discrepancy; the supervisee may lose confidence in you and become less willing to be open and honest as they perceive your interest as feigned.

Some plausible supervisee statements about genuineness

'She just seems to be herself.'
'I trust her to be honest with me.'
'I never feel misled by what she says.'
'She is genuinely pleased to see me.'
'She will show her feelings to me when it really matters.'

Acceptance (or warmth)

Gilmore (1973) has described acceptance as *'celebrating the diversity and complexity of human beings'*, so I feel this quality can be grouped in with the core conditions. If a supervisee can experience acceptance then they begin to trust the supervisor more and feel safe to continue to explore their own thoughts and feelings. If the supervisee is denied acceptance and positive regard, or if these things are made conditional upon certain aspects of behaviour, for example by being judged and criticized unnecessarily, so the supervisee may begin to lose touch with what their own experience means for them. As the above definition implies, acceptance is also about valuing each individual and their own uniqueness. For the supervisor, it is about recognizing both positive and negative aspects of the supervisee and a wholehearted willingness to work with them. It does not mean, however, agreeing with everything they may say or do: there will be times to challenge actions and behaviours that are self-defeating, unproductive, uncaring or against ethical principles of practice. By being accepting you will be creating a relationship that will feel sufficiently safe for the supervisee to feel cared for while exposing the more negative aspects of their work. Consider acceptance as an attitude towards the supervisee, recognition of how they are thinking or feeling and that they are being heard and understood. Acceptance and also warmth in a relationship can be conveyed and expressed through non-verbal as much as verbal communication, for example by eye contact, facial expression and tone of voice. Think of someone who is genuine in their warmth and acceptance towards you. Ask yourself how they demonstrate this by their non-verbal communication.

Acceptance is among the first steps of creating the safe and trusting supervision relationship. With acceptance, the supervisee is more likely to explore and expose the issue further, be more open to challenge and self-challenge (Inskipp 1996). Acceptance means that you are not asking questions of them.

Beware also of saying things like 'if I were you, I would' and 'yes, but don't you think.' Such responses are probably saying 'if you were me'.

Example of accepting and non-accepting responses

Supervisee: I just can't take much more at work. I started out with the best of intentions on that ward, but everyone seems so negative about the changes that are about to take place.

Supervisor: [Non-accepting] Give it a while longer, I am sure things will settle down.

Supervisor: [Accepting] You sound rather frustrated with the situation at the moment and you're wondering how long you will stay positive?

Whereas the non-accepting response ignores the supervisee's feelings, the accepting response demonstrates that you have heard what is being said. It communicates empathy by acknowledging the feelings and encourages further talking. This skill is called paraphrasing and is among several active listening skills that can be used to communicate acceptance and the other core qualities.

Unconditional positive regard (or respect)

Unconditional positive regard (UPR) means that the supervisor accepts the supervisee unconditionally and non-judgementally. The supervisee feels free to explore all thoughts and feelings, positive and negative, without danger of rejection or disapproval. Also, crucially, the supervisee does not have to earn the right to gain the positive regard of the supervisor. Rogers (1961) first described this concept as warm caring and acceptance for the client. It sets no conditions on the thoughts, feelings or behaviour of the individual; it is not possessive, nor does it demand any personal gratification in return. Sanders (1994) points out that these conditions can bring about potential areas of conflict for a counsellor when there is a genuine dislike of or distaste for what someone has done. Potential dilemmas can also arise when you strongly disagree with the actions and behaviour of your supervisee, for example in relation to their attendance and use of the clinical supervision sessions. You do have your supervision contract to fall back on regarding issues of breaking any supervision agreement. You will be required to give honest feedback and make judgements in such circumstances. This needs, however, to be respectful. Remember, you are giving judgements and feedback on their behaviour, not on them as a person. Sanders (1994: 58) writes: '*Seeing someone as worthy does not mean that you have to approve of their behaviour.*'

There may be more serious issues disclosed regarding unsafe or unethical practice or any illegal behaviour that concerns you. This may call for you to change your hypothesis of unconditional positive regard to one of conditional positive regard. You will need to discuss your concerns and thoughts on these matters first with the supervisee. This needs to be done, however, with respect, sensitivity and professionalism. If they are unwilling to take it through the appropriate organizational procedures then it will be your responsibility to do so. Remember that as practitioners you are both bound by the NMC code of professional conduct (2008). I raise these issues here as it can cause conflict for your genuineness and demonstration of unconditional positive regard. It will no doubt call for soul searching and being honest with yourself. I suggest that rather than turning your back on becoming a supervisor, you should view such circumstances, if they were ever to arise, as a positive challenge and more importantly for the benefit of patient care. It does highlight again the need for your own continuing support from your supervisor, manager, educator and organization. It also highlights the value of developing an honest and trustworthy relationship from the beginning with your supervisee in really getting to know each other as people as well as practitioners.

Some plausible supervisee statements about UPR

'No matter what, I always feel I am respected.'
'Whatever I say or do, at times she remains the same towards me.'
'When I have been in a bad mood it does not seem to affect the way she is towards me.'

How do we develop the personal qualities of being more empathic, accepting and genuine?

Most people that work in the helping professions will have the necessary core qualities in various degrees and measures. Taking your first steps into a supervision relationship will involve developing these qualities at a deeper level. Some suggestions for helping with this are listed below:

- Think of someone you know well; imagine standing in their shoes. How might they describe you?
- Your boss is writing a reference for you as clinical supervisor. What might they say about your helping qualities?
- When meeting new people in your life, take some time out to think about the similarities and differences. Which is the easier or more difficult to be empathic with, the similar or the different person?
- Talk to someone (or a small group) whom you feel safe with and trust. Explore some of your assumptions about and attitudes towards people in general.
- Listen to the others with an open mind. How different are their perceptions?
- How accepting are you of yourself? Both the positive and negative aspects.

- Ask yourself, 'How self-aware am I?' And, as regards helping qualities, 'What do I need to work on?'

How do we communicate these qualities?

It is a step in the right direction to develop these qualities for the supervision relationship. The important next step is to communicate them when we are supervising. The active listening skills of reflecting, paraphrasing and summarizing are among the key skills needed to do this; they are elaborated on in Chapter 5.

Self-awareness and the clinical supervisor

In order to build a supervision relationship based on the core conditions you will need to be more fully able to understand and recognize your true thoughts and feelings. This will require development in self-awareness.

You would think that with all the genius and the brilliance of this world we are living in, there would be a true and defined method to help us become self-aware. Well, I have not discovered one yet, so I guess I will have to look within myself. The ancient Chinese philosopher Lao Tzu is quoted as saying: *'He who knows others might be wise but he who knows himself is enlightened.'* I believe that we cannot entirely become self-aware and it is not an easy task to achieve. Stein-Parbury (1993) proposes that it can take a long time and that it is dynamic, not static. Let us now consider some ways and means of becoming more self-aware and its value to you as a supervisor. There is a vast amount of literature in the helping professions on the value of self-awareness in nursing and allied health professions (see, for example, McCabe and Timmins 2006).

Burnard (1992) gives six reasons why self-awareness is necessary for health-care workers:

- To enhance self-understanding.
- To allow self-acceptance of others.
- To enable us to handle difficult situations.
- To increase conscious use of self.
- To enable self-monitoring.
- To enhance personal autonomy.

Reflective activity

With those six reasons in mind:

- Think of a recent encounter in the work setting where your self-awareness enhanced and enabled your capacity to deal with the situation.
- What did you learn about yourself that was positive?
- Knowing what you do now, think of an encounter in the work setting when a lack of self-awareness resulted in not dealing with the situation as well as you might have done.
- What did you learn about yourself that was negative?
- Does this still occur?
- As a clinical supervisor, what aspects of your self-awareness will enhance and enable your practice?
- What aspects of self may hinder your practice?
- Comparing the positives and negatives about ourselves can be valuable in developing self awareness. True or false?

Using the analogy of the emotional bank account (Covey 1992) that was offered in Chapter 2, we might relate to the notion that most relationships can fluctuate greatly depending on what you invest emotionally and give of yourself. As a supervisor, being self-aware and keeping healthy the balance of the relationship is a responsibility you will have as part of the overall agreement.

As Rogers (1980) proposes, the core conditions, if they are to be truly effective, need to be incorporated into the person's way of being. You may like to think of them becoming an inside job, so to speak. I mean here that they originate and manifest from within, they become part of your own core self and part of your spirit. The principles of the core conditions need to become a fundamental belief and espoused as a way of being in all areas of helping relationships. As a supervisor, you carry the spirit of those qualities into the supervision relationship with you. They are not just taken down from the shelf when you enter the room and put back when you leave. Any attempt to use these qualities merely as a technique would soon be experienced by the supervisee as inauthentic and would prevent any worthwhile supervisory relationship from occurring. It can, however, be a difficult requirement if we do not feel fully connected to ourself or the supervisee. We may need to develop greater self-awareness, which is also an inside job.

With increased self-awareness you will be more able to:

- Understand, know and accept what you are thinking and feeling.
- Label your feelings.
- Understand why sometimes feelings 'take over' and know what makes you angry, upset or take on resentment.
- Understand that the way you think affects the way you feel, and how you feel can affect the way you think.

- Acknowledge that your thoughts and feelings influence your behaviour and decisions.
- Understand and recognize conflicting emotions and handle them in ways that are appropriate.
- Understand and use your knowledge and experience of how you think, feel and respond to choose your own behaviour, to the benefit of others, to learn and in particular build a positive relationship with your supervisee.

A self-awareness framework

A main feature of clinical supervision is to create an environment in which the supervisee has the opportunity to evaluate, reflect and develop their own clinical practice (Winstanley 2003). Self-awareness will be key to this process as it a vital component of learning and development (Burnard 1992). A good and popular framework to illustrate the usefulness of this process of self-discovery is the one devised by Joseph Luft and Harry Ingham (Luft 1969) which is commonly and affectionately referred to as the Johari Window (Figure 3.1).

OPEN AREA (1)	BLIND AREA (2)
Known by you and known by others	Unknown by you; known by others
'I am aware of my strengths and weaknesses, and so are you'	'I do not see the strengths and weaknesses about myself, but others do'
HIDDEN AREA (3)	UNKNOWN AREA (4)
Known by you; unknown by others	Unknown by you; unknown by others
'I see these aspects of myself but keep them hidden'	'Buried and a mystery to myself and others'

FIGURE 3.1 The Johari Window.

Put simply the Johari Window is a concept for understanding awareness in human behaviour and offers a way of looking at how personality is expressed. Freud and many others believed that we are only partially aware of our behaviour and that much of what we communicate is unconscious and non-verbal. If that is true then it has huge implications for healthcare workers and their interactions with clients. Self-awareness can therefore be seen as pivotal to both intra- and interpersonal relationships, and the model can be applied to any human interaction.

The Johari Window has four panes (or areas) as seen in Figure 3.1. They represent the following:

1 **Open area.**
   In everyday life: Is that part of our conscious self – our attitudes, behaviour, motivations, values, appearance, way of life – that we feel free and open

about and choose to exchange and share with others. The area increases in size as the level of trust increases, enabling more sharing of information.

In supervision: The supervisor shares this area willingly and their own view of their strengths and weaknesses is similar to the views of others.

2 Blind area.

In everyday life: Contains things that others observe about us that we do not know about; or things that that we imagine or perceive to be true of ourselves but that others do not see at all. To put this another way: aspects of ourselves that we are unaware of or aspects about which we are deluded. This will inevitably affect the way others act towards us. The blind area is very important in terms of personal development. How can we learn about ourselves and gain this information?

Unfortunately there is no ready answer but we can gain from putting ourselves in appropriate situations, where supportive and constructive feedback is invited and offered in a non-judgemental way. We need, however, to be open to feedback, to learn from others and to be open to change.

In supervision: The supervisor lacks a degree of insight into how others see their strengths and weaknesses. It suggests that we are unaware of certain mistakes that we keep repeating and do not recognize our potential to be more effective. Rogers (2004) uses the phrase '*bull in a china shop*' to describe a person for whom the blind area dominates.

3 Hidden area.

In everyday life: Represents things I know about myself and, for whatever reason, decide to hide from others. Strong emotional feelings towards others or secret thoughts and hidden messages that we retain out of fear are examples. The degree to which we can trust and then share ourselves with others (disclosure) is the degree to which we can be known. Confusion and misunderstanding in relationships can be reduced by being more open and honest with others

In supervision: The supervisor may feel inadequate and hide behind a facade. This can be exhausting as it takes a lot of energy to hide (Rogers 2004). Your supervisee may begin to perceive you as not genuine, which will probably result in a lack of trust and genuineness in the relationship.

4 Unknown area.

In everyday life: Contains things that nobody – including ourselves – knows about us; they are beyond our present awareness or buried deep in the subconscious (repressions, unsolved conflicts, unpleasant experiences). This area becomes 'known' when we have sudden or unexpected insights or learning opportunities to discover aspects of ourselves that have been influencing intra and interpersonal relationships all along.

In supervision: During supervision, in particular if the relationship is creative and fully functioning, some aspects of the unknown may present themselves to both parties on deeper reflection and feedback.

The ideal for the supervisor, using the concept of the Johari Window, is one where the open area is considerably larger than all the others. Change to this area will affect and reduce the size of the other areas. This can be achieved by:

- Asking for, and then taking on board, feedback to reduce the size of the blind area.
- Honesty and taking risks of self-disclosure appropriately.

It is through feedback and disclosure that our open area can be enlarged, thus reducing the size of the other areas. We can then gain access to the potential within us, represented by the unknown area (Figure 3.2).

OPEN AREA (1)	BLIND AREA (2)
Known by you and known by others	Unknown by you; known by others
'I am more aware of my strengths and weaknesses, and so are you'	'I am becoming more aware of my strengths and weaknesses through being open to feedback, and am still willing to learn'
HIDDEN AREA (3)	UNKNOWN AREA (4)
Known by you; unknown by others	Unknown by you; unknown by others
'I am more open and less defensive; I take appropriate risks and disclose my thoughts and feelings'	'I continue to learn and develop, which opens up the potential to be more effective as a supervisor and a person'

FIGURE 3.2 Johari Window applied to supervision

In summary, the Johari Window is a model both of self-awareness and of communication. It is a very useful learning aid and analytical framework in understanding ourselves in relation to how others see us, thus creating the potential for richer and more rewarding relationships.

Reflective activity

1. Open	2. Hidden
Positive aspects of self	Positive aspects of self
3. Open	4. Hidden
Negative aspects of self	Negative aspects of self

Divide a large piece of paper into four boxes, as shown in the diagram. Write down in **box 1** your attributes, skills and qualities that you would describe as positive and that you like about yourself. These are aspects that you would be open about, known to you and known to others. Aspects of yourself that you would take into a supervision relationship.

In **box 2**, write down further aspects about yourself that are positive. These are perhaps attributes that you keep hidden and hold back from owning. They may be still developing and as yet have not reached their potential.

In **box 3**, write down your traits that you think are negative; the things that you do not like about yourself. They are known to you and often to others that know you. You are aware that you possibly could take them into a supervision relationship.

Now for **box 4**. Write down – or you may just want to keep these in your thoughts – your negative traits; those that you keep mainly hidden. You would choose carefully to whom you would disclose these. You may not wish to recognize some of these, but if you were really honest with yourself, what purpose do they serve you? How do they hold you back from reaching more of your potential? You would not like to think that you would take them into a supervision relationship. This box is understandably the most difficult, but it could deliver up the most rewards.

Now look at all four of your boxes.

- Which traits and attributes stand out first and foremost for you?
- Of the positives, which do you wish to develop?
- How might you achieve this?
- Of the negatives, which do you need to be the most open and honest about?
- How might you begin to let go of these?
- How can you develop your self-awareness?
- What have you learnt about yourself from this exercise?
- Whom would you share this with? Why?
- Whom wouldn't you share this with? Why not?

This self-awareness exercise corresponds to the Johari Window as you have been reflecting on both the open and the hidden areas of self. It might be a contradiction to say you have uncovered some blind areas, but even so, you may have some idea of what these aspects are. You may have had feedback in the past that you have turned a blind eye to and maybe even denied to yourself. If you were to recognize these defects of character it may be possible to say goodbye to them. They perhaps have served you well, but you now want to move on in your development. They may cease to serve you now if you strive to be genuine and self-aware in a healthy supervision relationship.

An aim in the supervision relationship is to help your supervisee to be more open and self-aware, to be able to disclose their hidden fears, feelings and thoughts that they feel uncomfortable with. Becoming more self-aware yourself and recognizing your own conflicts with self can enable empathic understanding. Therefore the Johari Window can be seen as an aid to communication between the supervisor and supervisee. You are both striving to be more open, less hidden and less blind in order to reach more of your potential.

Giving constructive feedback

The giving of constructive feedback is essential, as the purpose of clinical supervision is to facilitate learning and help change behaviour.

A supervisor's role is to offer and give feedback. Feedback is also a way to learn about ourselves and discover some of those blind areas that we looked at in the Johari Window. According to Power (1999: 86), *'the process of giving feedback is the stock in trade of the clinical nurse supervisor'*. Remember also that perhaps not many other people are willing to offer good constructive feedback to your supervisee on a consistent basis. You may even find that you are the only one who can, and that they value your feedback the most.

Perhaps not consciously, as it can be scary, giving feedback can be one of the main reasons that healthcare workers seek out supervision. This is because giving constructive feedback to the supervisee is a valuable way for the supervisor to learn more about themselves and the effect their role as a healthcare worker has on others. In summary feedback:

- Increases self-awareness.
- Offers options and greater choice.
- Offers opportunities for modifications and change.
- Encourages professional and personal development.
- Allows you, as a supervisor, to be aware of your motivation for giving feedback and that it is for the above reasons.

Guidelines for effective feedback to the supervisee

- Give all types of feedback constructively, as the aim is to enable the supervisee to learn and improve.
- Start with a positive; offer constructive comments on areas for development; end with a strength and on a positive note. This is often referred to as the feedback sandwich.
- Personalize feedback by using I statements such as 'I feel that', 'In my opinion'.
- Give feedback in small amounts; keep it brief.
- Be sensitive to the supervisee's feelings, self-esteem and reactions.
- Be clear, concise and specific; avoid generalizations.
- Refer to performance and behaviour that the supervisee has the capacity to change.
- Offer hints, alternatives and suggestions.
- Indicate the possible impact on the supervisee's productivity in the healthcare setting.
- Use dialogue, so the supervisee has the opportunity to clarify.

- Motivate and empower through encouragement to consolidate strengths and address limitations.
- Check that what you intended to say has been heard.
- Allow the supervisee time to discuss, seek clarification and, more often than not, the choice of whether to act on it.
- Ask for feedback on your feedback: 'Has this been helpful?', or 'What may have been more helpful?'
- Make feedback regular and a feature of most, if not every, session.
- Think of what your feedback says about you as a supervisor.

Source: Adapted from Egan 2002

Giving feedback to, and also receiving feedback from, your supervisee will produce the most benefit if it is regular and balanced. Balanced feedback refers not only to the amount of positive and negative but also to the fact that it must be balanced over a period of time and meet the needs of the supervisee. Power (1999: 99) recommends that feedback is *'to maintain a balanced blend of comment, instruction, advice and facilitated reflection, depending, of course on the needs of the supervisee'*. Pendleton et al. (1984) propose that we learn faster and better if positive aspects are described first and then move into constructive exploring.

Feedback can be given in a variety of ways. It can be immediate and specific to an issue or situation the supervisee is discussing. It should also be given at regular intervals as an overall evaluation of strengths and areas to develop over time. Keep feedback brief and to a specific point in relation to the behaviour; other points can be given later at the relevant times. Challenge and give feedback on present behaviour, as though you are offering a gift for the person's learning, for future development and change.

Giving too much feedback at once can overload, cause confusion and be a waste of time. By getting to know your supervisee you will be better able to judge when they are ready for feedback: for example, do they ask or do they tend simply to wait for your comments. As a general rule, it is useful first to ask the supervisee how they felt they performed in a certain situation, rather than going straight in with your own feedback.

Inviting the supervisee to give their own feedback

Here are some questions you might ask when the supervisee has been describing an incident:

- 'What did you think your strength was in dealing with that incident?'
- 'What pleased you most?'
- 'I'm wondering how you saw yourself in that situation?'
- 'In what particular ways do you feel you could have acted differently?'

These are open questions and reflective in their intention. They invite the supervisee to explore their own views and gain the most benefit from the question. They can also have the benefit of reducing any anxiety that might be there and therefore encourage the supervisee to be more open and receptive to your feedback.

Inviting yourself to offer feedback

The following examples can be used as a way of asking the supervisee whether they would like you to offer some feedback on what they have been saying:

- 'We have been talking about that particular client rather a lot recently and how you feel stuck when he begins to disclose his feelings. While you were describing that, I had some thoughts.'
- 'Would you like me to give you some feedback, because I was thinking something a bit different?'
- 'Would you mind if I made one or two observations on what you have just been talking about?'

The above examples also have the effect of creating a dialogue for the feedback through the session and gives you both opportunities to clarify, discuss and ask for suggestions. Think of feedback as a wheel that continues to move the relationship forward and in the right direction to meet its aims and objectives.

More hints and tips when giving feedback

Ask for the supervisee's reactions to your feedback. For example:

- 'Was what I said helpful?'
- 'In what way?'
- 'Was that the type of feedback you wanted?'

Personalize your feedback and use 'I' messages rather than 'you' messages. For example, 'I observe you as' and 'I experience you as', not 'you are' or 'you always'. Beginning with 'you' messages can be heard as an attack and lead to a defensive response. 'You always arrive late and in a rush' can be more appropriately rephrased as, 'I am rather puzzled because I have noticed you are sometimes late, as though you have had to hurry here.' Another example would be, 'You are very dismissive when talking about him'. Rephrase this as, 'I find you do use rather flippant comments at times when describing that person. I'm left wondering what's going on for you when that happens.' The 'I' messages here aim to be less judgemental and the comments are more focused and concise rather than generalizing.

Endeavour to make negative feedback constructive by offering it in such a way that your supervisee can learn and improve. You may want to think of yourself as a coach not a critic. Focus on what can be realistically changed and what is of value to the supervisee.

An example of immediate feedback with some of the guidelines in mind is as follows. In this scenario, the supervisee is unsure whether to apply for promotion and has been talking in a negative way about their ability. The supervisor may respond as follows:

> *Supervisor:* I feel you have the required experience, and, yes, you have some important decisions to think about. From my observations you are capable, motivated and, most importantly, well respected by your colleagues and patients. However, if I am honest, you do undervalue yourself. I find that perhaps you are your own worst enemy at times when you talk negatively about yourself. You have made moves before and have experience of interviews. Would it be helpful to focus on some of the attributes you have?

Reflective activity

An exercise in giving feedback to yourself

This exercise is a variation of one I often use in training, the aim being to practise the skills of giving constructive feedback using the guidelines that have been suggested. You will need paper and pen to take notes. There are separate stages.

Stage 1

Reflect on recent scenarios in your work setting when you have been in the role of helper. This could be with patients/clients, students, colleagues, relatives, carers or other healthcare professionals. Recall one incident in which you felt you performed well and in which the outcomes were positive, and another in which you felt you had limitations and in which the outcomes were more negative.

- Note down your strengths, skills and attributes used in both scenarios.
- Note down what and how you could have performed differently, in particular in the second scenario.

Stage 2

Referring to what you would have done differently, ask yourself the following:

- Would this be realistic?
- What might the consequences have been?
- What would you suggest that you do next time?
- Would there have been an alternative way?
- How might you put this into your practice? How might you achieve this?
- How would you know?

- What strengths do you have that motivate and empower you to learn and develop?

Imagine observing yourself in those two scenarios. Give yourself some constructive feedback, bearing in mind the guidelines in this chapter. How would you deliver this to yourself? You might want to try giving your feedback out loud, to practise the skills and guidelines, for example the feedback sandwich, being specific, referring to what you can realistically change and a suggestion as to how this might be achieved.

You could end the exercise by giving feedback to yourself and how well you gave feedback.

Following on from a session in which you have given feedback to a supervisee, take a little time to reflect and to ask yourself:

- What did I learn about myself as a supervisor? As a person?
- What did I learn about my supervisee?
- What do I need to keep in mind for the next meeting?
- What did I learn about giving feedback?

Conclusion

This chapter has focused on the importance of developing and sustaining a healthy clinical supervision relationship, the rationale being that the core conditions are considered essential to building a trusting and empathic relationship. The reasons to cultivate self-awareness as a supervisor have been highlighted in conjunction with some skills and techniques for giving constructive feedback. Some foundations are now in place for the relationship to commence. The next chapter explores a conceptual framework for the functions and tasks of clinical supervision.

Key learning points

- By understanding the value that the core conditions have for the supervision relationship the supervisor can begin to build and sustain a healthy relationship.
- Acknowledging the key principles of person-centred theory will enable the supervisor to help the supervisee to reach more of their potential, both in supervision and in their healthcare practice.
- A supervisor who values self-awareness for personal and professional growth is more likely to develop their own potential for the tasks and roles they carry out.

- A skilled and self-aware supervisor can genuinely communicate the core conditions for the benefit of creating a prosperous and healthy relationship.
- Establishing a healthy relationship with the underpinning principles of the core conditions will mean that the supervisor can more effectively and skilfully give regular, balanced and constructive feedback to the supervisee.

4

Three Functions of Clinical Supervision

Chapter outcomes

By reading this chapter, doing the reflective activities, and integrating the material into your supervision practice, you should be able to:

- Understand the importance and value of a conceptual framework for clinical supervision.
- Recognize and acknowledge distinct features and tasks of the normative, formative and restorative functions of clinical supervision.
- Recognize and acknowledge similarities between the three functions.
- Know about and possess some skills of the normative, formative and restorative functions of clinical supervision.
- Acknowledge the concept of support and challenge for the clinical supervision relationship.
- Recognize some key issues and skills to assist when a supervisee needs to change supervisor.

Introduction

In the context of clinical supervision, the terms 'normative', 'formative' and 'restorative' are now generally recognized and accepted as describing the functions that underpin the tasks of supervision. I introduced these concepts in Chapter 1, and it is now my intention to consider them more comprehensively. Often known as Proctor's model (see Proctor 1986), it is probably more

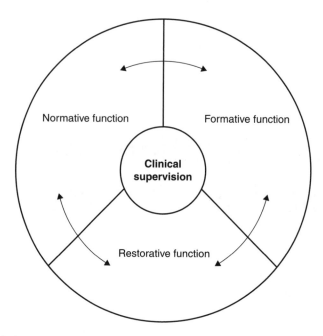

FIGURE 4.1 A conceptual framework for clinical supervision

appropriate to refer to it as a conceptual framework. The framework emerged from Proctor and her colleagues' work and experience in training and consultancy. It developed over the years and is now widely referred to in literature and training (Inskipp and Proctor 1995). Think of the framework as functions and overlapping components for the purpose of supervision. The three functions are evidence based, stemming from the history and literature of clinical supervision in a variety of healthcare contexts. Put simply, these three functions represent the three main aspects of clinical supervision and the three ways supervision can be offered to the supervisee. As stated earlier, they constitute a conceptual framework (Figure 4.1).

During clinical supervision the focus of the dialogue is on the issues raised in everyday working practice, with the aims and objectives of supervision being the task to achieve. The conceptual framework enables the supervisor to conceptualize, or in other words, to determine how and where to focus on the issues that the supervisee is bringing to the session, with those three functions in mind.

It is valuable to have this conception of supervision as it both guides and helps all parties involved as they work towards what they are trying to achieve. An understanding of the three functions also helps the supervisor to be aware

Three functions of clinical supervision

Normative. Within this function the supervisor is providing quality control, as they are enabling the supervisee to examine their work and to become more responsible in their own monitoring and maintenance of good standards of practice and adherence to policies. The supervisor recognizes (or, more accurately, shares with the supervisee) the responsibility for ensuring that the supervisee's work is ethical and professional and is operating within the norms, codes, laws and rules that the organization applies.

Formative. This function concerns and helps to form the development of skills, knowledge, attitudes and abilities by encouraging reflection on, and exploration of, the supervisee's work. The supervisor provides facilitation, feedback or direction to enable the supervisee to develop those attributes, so the supervisee becomes an increasingly competent practitioner.

Restorative. This function provides the support element. The supervisor accepts the supervisee as a human being in how they respond emotionally to the stresses and demands of working in the healthcare environment. The supervisor is restoring the supervisee when needed and is concerned with nurturing and affirming the supervisee and their overall well-being while practising in their work role.

of keeping an equal balance and the right kind of balance, which will depend on the needs of the supervisee and the issues being discussed. As a conceptual framework, it does not have a beginning or an end point, neither does it have stages to move through, so the framework is not prescriptive. The clinical scenario that is brought to the session by the supervisee may very well influence the starting point.

Reflective activity

- In what ways will your knowledge and understanding of this framework help and inform you as a supervisor when you begin clinical supervision?
- Reflect on your most recent clinical supervision session, either when you were giving or receiving. Ask yourself if the session contained elements of the three functions, or were one or two functions more prominent.
- What might some of the limitations be in using this framework as a focus for your supervision sessions?

I next consider each of the three functions in more depth, and look in particular at some skills, qualities and attributes that will be required.

The normative function

There is a certain amount of responsibility upon you, the supervisor, to ensure that the work of the supervisee is appropriate, competent, ethical, and meets the norms of their clinical area and profession. Although you are not responsible for their clinical practice, for example you are not acting as line manager, there is some responsibility that you carry. As the focus of the normative function is on maintaining appropriate standards of care and safe practice, there needs to be clear agreement of your responsibilities in the supervision contract. You will also need to have in place an agreed line of communication with their line manager or significant others, in the event that such issues do arise. You are assuming some form of management of the supervisee and need to be both comfortable and competent in this role. There is a range of approaches to employ in this role as there are several roles you may find yourself in. For example, you may need to be very prescriptive and strongly advise the supervisee on a certain issue, or you may need to be more exploratory and perhaps merely suggest action to take on a different issue.

Figure 4.2 shows a range of supervisory styles and approaches that can be used when the focus of supervision is in the normative mode. At the top of the continuum I have placed advising, and at the bottom exploring. There are also many types of intervention that can be used within each approach, for example you can give hard advice or soft advice.

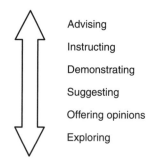

Advising

Instructing

Demonstrating

Suggesting

Offering opinions

Exploring

FIGURE 4.2 Supervisor style of normative interventions

Reflective activity

- Think of other styles that may be appropriate when in the normative mode, and where you would place them on the continuum in Figure 4.2.
- What would be some normative elements of your supervisee's work and practice?
- What issues might they bring to supervision or may arise?

- What style of normative interventions would you employ?
- Would you feel confident, comfortable and flexible using a range of normative interventions?
- Which style in particular do you need to develop?

Interventions that are generally more towards the exploratory end of the continuum would be more relevant to help the supervisee consider, act on and adhere to principles and practice that would fall in the normative function. Adults learn best when they feel free to direct themselves and can discover for themselves through the process of enquiry (Knowles 1984). There will, however, be need for flexibility in approach and style as you move back and forth on the continuum depending on the supervisee, the circumstance and issue. There may be issues that arise when you do need to be didactic, for example where safety procedures have been breached and you do need to make it very clear what action you, or they, or both of you will take. There will be occasions when you do need to be prescriptive and step in and say, 'I feel very strongly that you should think on that some more, for these reasons'. When there is more ongoing opportunity for reflecting on quality of care and developing standards for practice, a softer prescriptive approach can be used: 'How about considering that in a different way?', or 'My view on that would be . . . What do you think?'

It needs to be pointed out that the normative function is of paramount importance when it comes to fulfilling your role and responsibility as a supervisor. Also of paramount importance is for the supervisor to build a successful relationship whereby the supervisee can talk freely about their work. I have often found, when working with new supervisees, that they begin by needing support and will talk endlessly about their role, colleagues and the system. Perhaps because they are unfamiliar in the supervisee role or are still establishing trust with you, there is some initial hesitancy to self-disclose about, or question, their own individual involvement and interventions with patients. There may well be a fear of exposing weaknesses and vulnerabilities regarding their quality of care and skills. Sharing at appropriate times about your own patient or client involvement can help reduce any insecurity they may have. Disclosing how you have questioned yourself in certain clinical situations or when you learnt from mistakes by talking them over with a supervisor will also build trust. When the supervisee hears you taking risks by self-disclosing, they are more likely to take risks with more of their own self-disclosure.

Good supervising and the normative function

A good supervisor has the following awareness, values and skills:

- Is able to supervise others after acquiring sufficient training and/or experience in supervision.

- Competence to supervise on the areas of the supervisee's practice.
- Recognizes that supervision is influenced by organizational, professional and personal factors. For example, pressure on time for supervision means that you need to manage the process efficiently.
- Demonstrates self-awareness, sensitivity, respect, openness and interest about diversity in all forms.
- Is consistent in approach, attitude and performance.
- Is well informed and able to maintain the norms of clinical supervision, for example keeping boundaries, confidentiality, record keeping, organizational agreements and keeping to the contract.
- Is well informed about the norms of the supervisee's practice setting, for example the codes of conduct and related ethical issues.
- Is able to model ethical behaviour in response to concerns that may arise.
- Can maintain equilibrium in the face of crises.
- Is comfortable with the role of supervisor, for example being in a position of responsibility and influence and being an authority figure.
- Is comfortable carrying out evaluative functions.
- Is reliable, for example arrives on time, finishes on time, is prepared to organize the venue and facilities.
- Is able to carry out any administrative duties associated with supervision.
- Can appreciate the dynamics of the supervision relationship.
- Is able to be assertive, confront, challenge and negotiate.
- Has a clear sense of own strengths and limitations as a supervisor.
- Is able to identify how and when strengths and limitations may affect the conduct of supervision.
- Is able to evaluate the supervisory process and has confidence in giving and eliciting constructive feedback.
- Has reliable backing and support from their manager/employer for their role, responsibilities and duties as a clinical supervisor.

The formative function

The focus of the formative function is on developing the knowledge and skills of the supervisee. Supervision is an opportunity for the supervisee to learn and for them to utilize and transfer that learning to the benefit and good of their work role and responsibilities. The amount of focus in the formative function will depend on your own experience and knowledge of your supervisee's healthcare setting and role. They may have chosen you because of your expertise and skills in the same or a similar clinical role. This will have its advantages, but remember it is their learning and development that is taking place and not a forum for you to teach and display all that you know. A disadvantage in being an expert in their field can be that your supervisee will always seek the answers from you, look up to you and, if you allow them, never feel they will become as good as you. If you are not from a similar clinical environment then it is important that this is recognized and your skill will be in enabling them to reflect more on their own learning and in directing them to people with whom, and to resources where, they can acquire more knowledge. You do not know, and are not expected to know, everything they may be seeking advice or information on. This is perfectly okay. It can even enhance connectedness to say 'I don't know' if you are then both to seek the answers elsewhere and return to share your findings.

I endorse the sentiments of Powell (2004: 173) when he talks about the unanswered question being a *'fine travelling companion'* and that *'supervisees don't care how much a supervisor knows until they know how much they care'*. However, there will most certainly be occasions when you will need to refer your supervisee to other resources for information outside of the supervision relationship: for example, when more expert advice and consultation is needed on specific circumstances such as when a client has disclosed sexual abuse to the supervisee; or when evidence-based knowledge related to a specific skill or technique is needed to change a policy or procedure; or when ethical issues and legal matters arise that require more expert guidance.

Good supervising and the formative function

A good supervisor has the following awareness, values and skills:

- Has enthusiasm for learning and development.
- Has understanding of adult learning.
- Is able to motivate and view motivation as a supervisory task.
- Has knowledge and skills of reflective practice.
- Is able to allow freedom of thought and expression.
- Can encourage and empower the supervisee to recognize and acknowledge own personal experience and growth.
- Can inspire the supervisee to develop and believe in own abilities.
- Maintains self and professional continuing development in own area of clinical practice.
- Has ability to show and teach new skills and techniques in the context of the supervisee's learning where applicable, or to refer to other resources to enable their development.
- Has ability to facilitate and encourage the supervisee to translate theory into practice, when appropriate, with emphasis on evidence-based material.
- Has ability to pace the learning and development to the supervisee's needs and requirements. Not too fast so they lose heart and not too slow so they stagnate.
- Has clear thinking, verbal expression and congruence and is able to bring clarity to confusion.
- Has analytical skills, problem identification skills and problem-solving skills.

- Is able to negotiate and develop agreement on goals and tasks when and where applicable.
- Has reliable links with an education provider regarding supervision training, issues and updates.
- Has a love of teaching and can achieve fulfilment by assisting the supervisee to develop more of their own potential.

It is important to recognize the learning needs and level of what is required for the supervisee's stage of experience and responsibility. The recently qualified supervisee or those new to their current role will have different requirements from those who have had considerable time in practice. These different requirements will determine your own level of functioning in this formative role. If your supervisee has considerable experience in a speciality, you will need to ask yourself how far you are able to help them develop in their role. There will come a time when a change of supervisor is going to benefit your supervisee if the formative function is to sustain itself. View this as positive for your supervisee and for yourself: you have fulfilled your role and now they are ready for a new challenge. A different perspective can offer a new challenge and experience for the supervisee's continuing professional development.

The restorative function

The focus of this function is to nurture and care for the well-being of the person being supervised, by creating a therapeutic relationship. Healthcare workers are often in contact with their patient's pain, personal distress, loss and anxiety, to name but a few of the emotions and disabilities that they face on a daily basis. This supportive function serves to help the worker acknowledge and work through their own feelings when affected by or caught up with the emotions and helping relationships they are engaged in. The supervisor's role is to facilitate exploration and release of feelings. This can help the supervisee to see things more objectively. By sharing some of the burden and becoming more rational in thinking, the supervisee may avoid becoming over-involved in others' distress, to the point where it affects their own well-being. While offering support and being supportive, it is important not to view this function as seeing deficits or weakness in the supervisee, or indeed their organization.

There needs to be a balance by focusing too on the joys and accomplishments of the supervisee. We do spend a lot of our waking hours at work, with perhaps not enough focus on the enjoyment that that can bring. So spend time talking about achievements and give praise and encouragement to continue in a similar manner. Help your supervisee to laugh and see the lighter side of life at times. Find ways to be creative and make the supervision enjoyable and healthy by balancing up with the more pleasurable aspects of the supervisee's work and professional relationships.

Reflective activity

Think about a supervisee you are working with. Consider and focus on the restorative aspects of their work.

- Do you have the necessary awareness of, and insight into, the demands of their role and work environment?
- In relation to their work role and patient–client contact, what may be the stressful and distressing features?
- What might the supervisee bring to supervision that would need your support?
- What do you feel they may be reluctant to talk about and why?
- What may be the joys, pleasures and achievements of their work?
- How do you generally give support to others in your work role?
- What further skills or techniques do you need to develop for this function?

It is all-important when being supportive to get to know your supervisee really well as a person and as a professional helper. What they find a stressor may be different from what you expect or what others in a similar role find stressful. So get to know them as an individual with individual needs and expectations. As you get to know your supervisee, you may become the first person to notice what tends to stress them the most and when they really do need support. You also may become the one person they trust enough to turn to when things are difficult. As you begin to recognize and become more aware of your supervisee's needs, you will need the skills to communicate that understanding to them and in particular the feelings they may be experiencing.

Develop a repertoire of feeling words

The use of active listening and attending skills is the basis of interventions in the formative function. These skills will be explored in some depth in Chapter 5. If we are to develop skills to reflect back feelings which are not being overtly expressed by the supervisee, we can be more accurate by increasing our vocabulary of feeling words. By becoming more emotionally literate we develop self-awareness and personal insight to more accurately examine our own feelings and to recognize feelings in others. Also, by developing our vocabulary of feeling words we enhance our ability to distinguish between different emotions and feelings. Stein-Parbury (1993) argues that a major difficulty in reflecting feelings is the limited language the helper possesses to describe them. Feelings are more subtle than emotions. The emotion of anger, for example, we would all have experienced and probably be able to recognize.

However, each of us would have a range of different feelings and experiences that we would use to describe that anger. Increasing our vocabulary can make a wider range of feeling words more accessible and enable us to reflect more accurately and empathically to that unique supervisee. This will also avoid the dialogue becoming mechanical or superficial and can enhance our ability to communicate genuineness and empathic understanding.

A popular exercise often used to increase our feeling vocabulary is included in the following reflective activity.

Reflective activity

- Recall a number of emotional situations at work and think of as many feeling words as you can to describe them.
- Use a thesaurus to look up synonyms for those words that express the emotion.
- Keep a notebook and write down feeling words you hear expressed by staff as they go about their daily work. Put them under headings or feeling categories, for example anger, fear, sadness, happiness, hope.
- You could also arrange the words along a continuum of mild, medium and strong intensity. I have suggested some feeling words below. Fill in the question marks with your own choice of words, as many as you can, that represents the feeling and the level of intensity.

	Mild intensity	Medium intensity	Strong intensity
Angry	?	?	Outraged
Fear	Uneasy	?	?
Sad	?	Miserable	?
Happy	Pleased	?	?
Hope	?	Optimism	?

Source: Adapted from Carkhuff 1983

When this exercise is performed in training groups there are many alternatives and not all people would agree on the subtle differences between intensity. We discover also that many feeling words contain feelings within them. With practice it becomes easier to indentify feelings from non-verbal as well as verbal communication, and by developing a repertoire we can choose our words to reflect back more accurately and empathically. It is important to note that when reflecting back feelings you should attempt to choose a word that is as close to the supervisee's feelings as possible. To overstate the feeling can result in the person backing away or wanting to change the subject. To understate or to be more accurate can help the person to express that feeling and elaborate more, as they are on more familiar ground, rather than the unknown.

Good supervising and the restorative function

A good supervisor has the following awareness, values and skills:

- Has faith in the task and process of supervision.
- Is nurturing, calm and generous in giving to others and self in supervision.
- Can listen attentively.
- Is non-judgemental, warm and congruent.
- Is able to have and to communicate empathic understanding.
- Is able to communicate compassion.
- Is able to integrate the spirit of supervision when supporting staff on an ongoing and regular basis.
- Is able to convey a positive, approachable attitude and personality.
- Has a sense of humour, which helps you both get through the rough patches and achieve a healthy perspective on your work together.
- Can convey and share the pleasurable aspects of work.
- Can introduce creativity when needed.
- Is able to admit to their mistakes.
- Has, and is developing, emotional intelligence.
- Can share time, knowledge and experience willingly, without expecting recompense.
- Ensures support for own self.

A vignette demonstrating the three functions of supervision

Ruby, a newly qualified nurse of several months, was very enthusiastic about her work and wanted desperately to do well in her career. At one session, Ruby arrived appearing rather anxious and looking tired. Tearfully she disclosed that family matters were causing distress for all concerned. The supervisor used active listening skills, e.g. open questions, reflecting, clarifying and appropriate silence, to communicate empathic understanding, to help her continue talking and to demonstrate support [**restorative**].

Ruby's parents, whom she lived with, along with two younger sisters, had been constantly arguing and disagreeing about another family member's decision to divorce their partner. This was a rather taboo subject within the family. Ruby felt it her responsibility to be peacemaker to her parents, whom she had only rarely seen disagree in the past. Her worst fear was that her parents may even separate. Following appropriate challenging by the supervisor [**restorative**] and allowing her to reflect on this, she felt that was extremely unlikely. She wanted to protect her sisters from the constant disputes. Subsequently she was spending a great deal of time with all the family members individually talking, placating and pacifying. Ruby was feeling tired, distracted and worried about her job.

Through further exploration and empathic listening [**restorative**], Ruby felt she had put herself in this role as she was a nurse who had helping skills and needed to do good and to make things better. However, she had barely made work on time, been late twice and was generally preoccupied. A member of staff had said she had better 'sort this out'. The supervisor asked her how she felt on hearing such comments and what she needed to do regarding her reliability at work [**normative**]. Ruby spoke of her current duties and responsibilities. She was aware of letting others down if this situation continued. The supervisor stressed the importance of exploring options to find a valid way forward that would enable Ruby to maintain the quality of her performance at work [**normative**] during this stressful time at home.

Through active listening, challenging and exploration [**restorative**], Ruby began to recognize that this family issue was not her responsibility and that her parents would not want it to be affecting her work, if indeed they knew. By encouraging and motivating [**restorative**] Ruby to focus on her quality of work [**normative**], the supervisor and Ruby together explored her assertive skills for use with her family and her time management skills for arriving at work, not only in good time, but also in a positive frame of mind [**formative**]. By helping Ruby to identify her personal and professional responsibilities [**formative** and **normative**] and to put them into practice [**formative**], Ruby was able to learn that the role she had taken upon herself at home was self-defeating [**formative**].

Having talked through this family matter that was causing her problems focusing on work [**restorative** and **normative**], Ruby was able to separate the two and learn new skills [**formative**] to help keep her focused. She was subsequently able to restore herself to be a fully functioning member of her work team once more [**normative**].

I have attempted with this vignette to demonstrate the focus and purpose of the interventions used in relation to the three functions. I chose the scenario to demonstrate that issues at home and with family can and do cause issues for work.

Reflective activity

- Reflect on your own supervision for your clinical practice and ask yourself: Overall, does your supervisor provide a balance between the three functions that can be identified as normative, formative and restorative, when you are discussing and reflecting on key issues? If not, why not?
- Reflect on a recent supervision session you have carried out and ask yourself: Are you able to identify working with the three functions during that session? (Use the vignette as an example.)

- Was there an equal balance determined by the session content?
- What do the three functions have in common?
- What differences are there?
- Reflecting on the three functions as a concept, ask yourself: Would you have done anything differently, and if so why?
- Which of the three functions do you most need to develop skill and technique in?

Generally, as a supervisor you need to be aware of having a balance of the three functions. However, this will depend on the nature of the issues being discussed. The restorative function can be said to underpin all sessions whereas the main and most important focus is on the normative function. During the process of offering support for the supervisee to focus on their practice and performance, the supervisee can learn and develop new skills as befits the formative function. Bond and Holland (1998) endorse this notion. They place the normative function at the heart of clinical supervision. For the supervisee to feel safe enough or able enough to discuss their clinical practice (normative) they need first to feel that they are to be supported (restorative) and that learning will be part of the process (formative). So it becomes that, through the restorative and formative processes, the normative aspects may be focused on and worked through, thereby fulfilling the central objective of clinical supervision: the well-being of our patients and aspects of quality care (Bond and Holland 1998).

A balance of support and challenge

Keeping your supervisee motivated to continue to learn and develop within all three functions, a good clinical supervisor balances the giving of support and challenge. It was Rogers's (1969) view that learning is most successful when motivation is high. Studies carried out by Martin (1996) and McNally et al. (1997) found that a combination of support and challenge was a key ingredient for growth, motivation and quality of learning. Although those studies focused on student teachers, there are many similarities that would advocate that supervisees, as learners themselves, also need the ingredients of support and challenge. Daloz (1986) designed a model of mentoring known as the support, challenge and vision model (Figure 4.3). As supervision is an ongoing relationship you need to remain both faithful and committed to the development of the supervisee, both during stable times and in the midst of change, growth or transition. To accomplish this I feel it is important to be faithful to Daloz's model and offer support, challenge and vision. I include the model here as a means to consider and understand your interactions and dynamics in

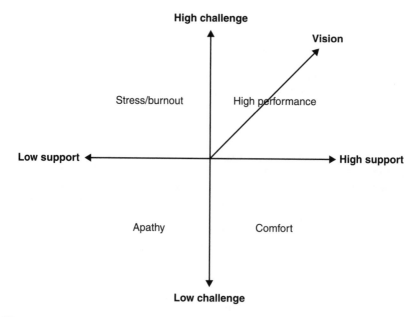

FIGURE 4.3 A balance of support and challenge

the development of your supervisees. View each of the four quadrants as positions for the support and challenge you offer your supervisee.

Each of the positions will be now be considered in turn.

Low support, low challenge

This position is most likely at the beginning of supervision when the supervisee is new. Now that they have ongoing and regular supervision, support can continue to develop. You are helping them to feel generally positive about themself and are demonstrating interest in their work. When you are taking your first steps, establishing the relationship and getting to know each other, this may often feel to be the starting point for the supervisee. The relationship, however, is your springboard to be able to give all the support and challenge the supervisee needs. If both support and challenge remain low then the supervision is very unlikely to foster productive learning experiences and will remain unsatisfactory for all concerned in the process. Stimulus to continue with supervision will also be low. To remain in this position can result in apathy.

High support, low challenge

This position is most likely when the supportive relationship has been established and the supervisee feels valued and respected. Supervision has become a safe place to talk and take risks. Any initial uncertainties and anxieties have been reduced. The supervisee has a strong sense from you that they are doing well enough and trust you as a good sounding board for ideas. There is a danger that this position can become rather comfortable, and, although their work is competent, further development in learning is not being stretched. If challenge remains low there may be a lack of motivation to develop professionally, unless the supervisee is self-motivating or has this requirement met elsewhere. On occasions you may need to stay in this context for a period of time, for example if the supervisee is a recently qualified practitioner who is still learning the ropes. They are perhaps discovering how little they do know, how much there is to learn, and will need high support. When the pressure is really on for your supervisee, or they are going through many difficulties, transitions or a leave of absence, they will also need a period of high support, low challenge. To remain in this position, however, can result in too much comfort for the supervisee.

Low support, high challenge

There may be specific occasions when this position has value. The supervisee is an accomplished practitioner; they have good supportive colleagues but need to be challenged on a particular aspect of their work. They request from you some high challenge for a period of time, although they are aware that support will be there from you as and when needed. Other than the above context, if the position were to continue in general then the supervisee might retreat to a comfort zone or face a downward spiral of motivation. It is also worth considering that your supervisee may often be in the position of low support and high challenge in their work environment and perhaps in other aspects of their life. Stress and burnout in the work situation can result if this position is prolonged.

High support, high challenge

Effective learning development takes place in this position and this is the most productive and conducive to the empowerment of the healthcare worker and professional growth. Overall, this is generally the dynamic to aim for in supervision. However, you need to recognize when the supervisee might be struggling and in danger of sinking, so that you can move back to giving high support and low challenge. Effective supervisors need to both balance and blend together these ingredients. By being highly supportive you have the supervisee's respect and have provided a safe place to be able to challenge the supervisee to push on and move forward. This position is one of high performance.

Vision

Vision refers to the ultimate goal of the high support, high challenge context: not only to achieve this dynamic but also to maintain and continue its progress. It is important to remember that:

- **Effective supervisors can successfully create this dynamic.**
- **Effective supervisors foster in the supervisee the vision and means to continue in their development of quality professional practice.**

Reflective activity

Refer back to Figure 4.3 and ask yourself the following:

- What words or comments would you put in each of the four quadrants when you have experienced that position in your work setting?
- At your current stage of development as a healthcare professional, what balance of support and challenge do you need from your supervisor?
- What could change that balance for you?
- Think of one of your supervisees. What balance of support and challenge is there?
- Are you able to recognize what different supervisees will need and when?
- How and with whom will you maintain your capacity, creativity, strength and skills to keep this vision in mind when providing clinical supervision?

Changing supervisors

Earlier in this chapter it was noted that a supervisee at some point in the future will benefit from a change of supervisor, in particular with the formative function in mind to further their personal and professional development. Moving towards that change can be arranged and worked through over time in a positive and professional way. However, a situation may arise requiring a supervisee to discontinue for other reasons. This can be the result of an unforeseen change in practical or organizational circumstances, or for a variety of other personal or professional reasons. First and foremost, remember the principles and spirit of supervision to address this. The concept of the three functions may also help you to attend to some of the issues together as you discuss ending the supervision relationship.

I offer some examples here of applying the three functions when the supervision relationship is unable to continue and a rather sudden ending is imminent.

- Normative: That you will both attempt to do this professionally and in the best interest of the supervisee, the organization and yourself.
- Formative: That you both take away any learning that you can.
- Restorative: That it is addressed with care and support.

The best possible way to achieve the above is to discuss face to face and arrange a session for this. If, for organizational reasons, the supervisee is unable to continue, then ensure that they are to leave feeling valued. Offer appropriate constructive feedback from their time with you and clear up any contractual issues, for example where any notes or records will go and who needs to be informed. Communicate enthusiasm and interest in their development and continued use and arrangements for supervision elsewhere.

If they have more personal reasons for wanting to change supervisor then here are some tips to employ:

- Listen to what the supervisee has to say and don't argue. The best way to manage conflict is to work it out between yourselves and reach a resolution that would suit you both.
- Supervision is about reflecting, ensuring standards, learning and supporting, so attempt to resolve the difficulties between you with that in mind.
- Refer back to, and review, your contract regarding rights and responsibilities and ask what changes need to happen if the relationship is to continue. Make any amendments as appropriate and if agreed. Negotiate and work together to resolve any issues that can help make the relationship and the supervision change for the better. Set a time in the near future to review this again.
- Terminating the contract with unresolved issues and conflicts can leave you both feeling bad and not knowing what went wrong.
- With the agreement of your supervisee, and perhaps as a last resort, arrange for a third party to meet with you both. This can help resolve the rather more complex issues regarding the relationship. Having an external facilitator can help you both see more objectively and reflect on the issues you are both caught up in. It will also put less pressure on you in being responsible for the outcome.
- It is important that you both learn and develop from the experience.
- Talk this through with your own supervisor first, and also afterwards.

The three functions and research

Cutcliffe (2001) cites how researchers can use the three functions of supervision in evaluating supervision's effectiveness. Among some of the early studies of whether supervision made a measurable difference to levels of stress in supervisees, the findings were certainly positive (Butterworth et al. 1997). Interviews with, and questionnaires completed by, healthcare workers revealed the value of supportive interventions and qualities that would fall within the restorative function. Identifying which of the three functions are more prevalent as themes that emerge during sessions could possibly be utilized for research purposes. Some further consideration is given to this in Chapter 9 when we look at evaluating clinical supervision sessions.

Conclusion

This chapter has focused on a conceptual framework that encompasses both the tasks and the functions of clinical supervision. Having knowledge and understanding of those tasks, the supervisor will need good communication skills in order to perform them in the most helpful manner. In the next chapter we look at active listening and responding skills, which are essential for the supervisor to begin this process.

Key learning points

- Being able to define and understand a conceptual framework for clinical supervision will help to keep the focus in mind for the overall aims and objectives of clinical supervision.
- Understanding the purpose of the normative, formative and restorative functions of clinical supervision the supervisor can more readily and competently meet the needs of the supervisee and the organization, with the overall intention of benefiting patient care.
- A skilled supervisor develops their skills and techniques of supervising within the normative, formative and restorative functions.
- A skilled supervisor understands that a balance of support and challenge are needed in enabling the supervisee to function at the optimum level.
- Recognizing that the concept of the three functions of supervision have an underpinning value and focus for the supervisor's own training and development as a supervisor.

5

Active Listening and Responding Skills

Chapter outcomes

By reading this chapter, doing the reflective activities and integrating the material into your supervision practice, you should be able to:

- Define active listening and responding.
- Value and recognize the importance of active listening for the supervisor.
- Appreciate the core principles of active listening.
- Recognize the importance of, and possess some skills for, non-verbal attending.
- Recognize the importance of, and possess some skills of active listening and responding.
- Acknowledge the value of silence as a listening skill.

Introduction

Of the main authors who have contributed to raising the awareness of active listening skills, Burnard (1998) is among many that have acknowledged that they are essential for the healthcare worker skilled in interpersonal communication. It is important first of all to acknowledge that there is a difference between active listening/responding and the more normal, everyday listening/responding. When we are actively listening, it is the only activity we are carrying out. Normally, while going about our daily duties we are often doing several things at once, having lots on our minds such as thinking about the next task, planning and organizing our work or having conversations and listening to others. Active listening is defined here as giving the other person your full concentration and sole attention while taking an active interest in them, for example when supervising.

It goes without saying that the benefits of active listening are greater effectiveness for you, for the supervisee and for the relationship. We demonstrate that we are genuinely interested in what the supervisee has to say. It is one of the most effective ways to express our acceptance and respect for the supervisee. They will feel more valued and that what they say as an individual really matters; they will then listen to you the more. By being a role model as a good listener you can also teach the supervisee how to listen. It would be a positive assumption that they go on to be a good listener in their other professional and personal relationships.

Supervision in this formal context takes on a whole new dimension compared with when it is given while performing other duties or at break times. That is not to say that informal and ad hoc encounters are of no value. As a supervisor with a formal arrangement you are now in a privileged and important position, one where you have the opportunity to actively listen, respond and give full value. The relationship will benefit as more active listening encourages the relationship to grow with further depth of dialogue.

Listening as a supervisor

As a supervisor we have many gifts, including two ears and one mouth, which is commonly interpreted as nature's way of telling us that we need to listen more than we speak. Over the years, and with a great deal of practice, I have found that I learn far much more by listening to others than by talking. I may not agree with all I hear but I am still learning about others and myself. However, when being supervised I need to talk, reflect on my practice and be listened to, and I will learn from the listening and responses from my supervisor. Thinking back to when I first was supervised, I was not so concerned with how much my supervisors would say or how much they knew, my concern was if I could be open with them, if they were someone whom I could trust and feel comfortable with, which at first is demonstrated by their active listening. As a supervisee, I want to be understood, as I am not always able to verbalize my thoughts and feelings in a fully coherent way. Most communication problems are a result of misunderstanding, so an effective supervisor must at first seek to understand. As a supervisor, if I am able to understand another's situation, to begin to think and feel in the way that they do, as much as that is possible to begin with, then I am much more likely to be able to help. This requires the supervisor to listen more and talk less; but having said that, we do need to verbally communicate that we are listening.

Listening to build an empathic relationship

The active listening skills described in this chapter need also to become accurate listening skills. It may help to develop the accuracy by considering these as a set of tools in your supervision toolbox. By becoming more familiar with and identifying specific skills and their intention, we will be more able to respond accurately. Moreover, we will be able not only to communicate that we have received and understood what is being said by this unique individual who is sitting with us, but also, essentially, to build an empathic rapport. The empathic relationship has been discussed in Chapter 3 along with the importance of developing this in supervision. These accurate listening skills are among the first steps in achieving basic empathy. Freshwater (2003) points out that if the helper can step into the other's world, albeit only briefly, then they become better able to relate to the other person: they can develop some partial awareness of their thoughts, feelings and intentions. This at first is achieved by active and accurate listening and responding. The supervisee will begin to experience the helper's empathic responding and be more ready and able to feel safe, trusting and willing to develop the relationship to fulfil its goals and intentions.

Listening with the three functions of supervision in mind

We need supervisor's ears to be able to fully listen to and understand the supervisee's experiences in clinical practice. While listening to those experiences we can categorize them and understand them within the context of the three functions of supervision. This will help to keep a focus on the functions' aims and to keep a healthy balance within all three. The three functions of supervision were introduced and identified in Chapter 1 and dealt with in more depth in Chapter 4.

- **Normative function.** You are listening to the issues of practice that are being raised and discussed with regard to standards of practice, accountability and quality of care, so you can help reflect, problem solve and offer guidance when and where appropriate.
- **Formative function.** You are listening to issues of practice with regard to identifying learning needs and the refinement of acquired skills for personal and professional development, so you can offer feedback and help cultivate reflective learning and opportunities to learn.
- **Restorative function.** You are listening to issues of practice where thoughts, feelings and emotions emerge with regard to the demands and pressures of working in a healthcare environment, so you can give support, nurturance, feedback and encouragement. You can also offer other forms of help or referral as appropriate.

Core principles for effective listening in supervision

Developing new habits, like many other endeavours in life, takes time, practice and patience. The way we listen is a habit. If we want to improve our communication skills, we will likely have to adjust our listening habits. This involves keeping some broad general principles in mind as you practise specific skills.

- Have a genuine desire to listen. Make sure you have time and are not tired.
- Have a feeling of trust in the other person's capacity to work out their feelings, make decisions and find solutions. Not only can we take responsibility for ourselves, but also we can allow others to take responsibility for themselves.
- Remember that people's feelings shift all the time. Feelings often change as a result of new information or insight.
- Avoid sharing your own stories and saying 'I know just what you are going through'.
- Remember the focus of the supervision session is not on you or about you; it is about the other person.
- The listening phase of a conversation means giving your complete attention to the speaker, not interjecting with your own concerns or experiences.
- Be patient, give space. You do have time to listen, so don't hurry.
- Practise letting the supervisee fully finish talking before planning your response. This may create periods of silence that may feel uncomfortable at first, but the person you're speaking to will soon learn to appreciate your desire to truly listen and your willingness to respond thoughtfully to their concerns.
- Develop a third ear to listen with. This means that you are listening attentively not only to what they are saying verbally but also to the subtext of their conversation. You are observing their overall body language, demeanour and posture, and making mental notes about what they might be going through.
- Learn to listen differently each time. Repeated issues and similar conversations that arise may sound familiar to you, but you can keep them fresh and gain new insights by listening differently each time.

Reflective activity

- From the above core principles, what would you find relatively easy to take into the supervision relationship?
- What would you find less easy?
- What other core principles of listening would you want to develop in a supervision relationship?

Non-verbal communication and listening

The basic skills that supervisors use involve listening, observing, attending and responding. These active listening skills require your full attention and alertness to what is being said as well as implied. We need first to consider and understand non-verbal communication, as it is among the foundations upon which human relationships are built (Okun 2002). It is often quoted that around two-thirds of communication is conveyed non-verbally. Further reading to support that theory can be found in the work of Michael Argyle (1994), a leading social psychologist in the field of interpersonal behaviour. There is extensive literature on the therapeutic value of communication skills for healthcare professionals, with evidence to support and improve practice (McCabe and Timmins 2006). In addition to the words we speak, very powerful messages are given in non-verbal communication (Thompson 2002). It is therefore important that supervisors focus on and analyse all their communication skills for their effective use in supervision. We all would like to think that we do employ and use good communication skills in our fields of practice. They have developed both naturally and through training and experience over time. Non-verbal communication is extremely difficult to avoid; it can be said that it is impossible not to communicate non-verbally with the person to whom we are talking. It is so commonplace that we can take it for granted and not be fully aware of the messages we are sending and how they may be influencing the interaction. We can, however, train ourselves to be more aware of this dimension of communication and its implicit messages. The influences it can have, however subtle they may be, can supplement our verbal helping skills in both positive and negative ways. But how often do we get feedback on the way we communicate, and in particular on our non-verbal communication?

Reflective activity

Reflect on the following non-verbal gestures possible while supervising:

Sitting with arms folded, sitting cross-legged.
Fiddling with a pen, folder or any other object that might be to hand.
Shuffling in your seat.
Scratching head or fiddling with hair.
Gazing out of the window.
Sneakily looking at your watch or the wall clock.
The telephone or your mobile starts to ring.
Finger pointing.
Gestures of disapproval, disgust, shock or even horror.

Imagine yourself as the supervisee:

- Which of the above would be off-putting to you?
- What might you read into these non-verbal barrier gestures?
- What kind of non-verbal messages would you want from your supervisor?

There are any number of things, consciously or unconsciously, that we can do during supervision sessions that may be off-putting to the supervisee. Most of the gestures listed in the above activity may indicate that we are not totally interested or that there is something else on our mind. The last two mentioned are among many gestures that imply being judgemental or allowing our own emotions to surface inappropriately. These and many other non-verbal barrier gestures can be insignificant and trivial to the supervisee; after all, your supervisee wants to see you as a real person who is not wooden and unnatural (in Chapter 3 we stressed the importance of demonstrating warmth and genuineness in the relationship). We do, however, need to be aware of when off-putting non-verbal communication has significance. Some behaviours we may be able easily to identify and consciously alter; others may be among our idiosyncrasies. Both types may be occasional or frequent. Self-awareness will help to raise our conscious use of self in this area of communication. Or you can ask a trusted colleague to give you feedback in a training or role-play situation. Remember, an aim of non-verbal communication in supervision is to enable the supervisee to feel they have been fully listened to and accepted.

Non-verbal attending

- **S**it squarely in front of the supervisee
- **O**pen body posture
- **L**ean slightly towards the supervisee
- **E**ye contact with the supervisee as appropriate
- **R**elaxed in posture

A useful mnemonic to remember is SOLER (Egan 2002), which identifies non-verbal behaviours for effective listening and attending (see the Box above).

This well-known and often cited mnemonic should not be read as the five commandments. For a variety of reasons, the five bodily positions may not all be possible throughout the session, and it will be quite natural to digress from them. Use SOLER along with the following pointers as a useful guide and attempt to retain or return to the features mentioned:

- I assume that you are not going to sit behind a desk. Position the seating fairly square on and at a distance that feels comfortable and non-threatening. The aim is to be face to face and in a position of equality, so avoid taking the best chair for a status symbol.

- Having an open body posture conveys that you are comfortable and open to whatever the supervisee has to say. Sitting with arms and legs crossed can be interpreted as being defensive, a reluctance to fully engage, or that you consider yourself in some way superior. Whom would you rather disclose something personal to, someone who has an open body posture, or someone who appears closed and not interested?
- Lean slightly towards your supervisee to indicate that you are interested and want to hear what they have to say. This may be uncomfortable and feel unnatural to do throughout the session, but attempt to maintain this position, especially when you sense your supervisee really wants your attention.
- Shakespeare wrote 'the eyes are the windows to the soul', and there are probably a thousand more metaphors that refer to the eyes. You can probably think of positive and negative ones without too much difficulty. What do you feel when you have been given a cold stare? How do you feel towards that person who only has eyes for you? We do communicate with our eyes, so eye contact needs to be positive and appropriate when communicating warmth, concern, trust, respect, interest and so on. A general rule is to keep eye contact gentle rather than intense (Cameron 2008). Aim to keep a balanced amount of eye contact, neither too little nor too much. Achieving an effective balance is not so easily done, especially when deciding what constitutes an appropriate balance. This may vary from person to person and according to culture, so self-awareness is required. Think about what raising of eyebrows may indicate: alarm at what has just been said or a sign that it is the other person's turn to talk?
- Last but not least is to be relaxed and to act naturally with all these aspects of non-verbal attending. If you do feel at ease, confident and comfortable with yourself in the role of supervisor then these will come more naturally.

Combining non-verbal cues with the spoken word

When non-verbal cues are used in combination with spoken words, the impact of the message is doubled. Knapp (1978) describes these impacts in the following way (note that the first two are positive, as the relevant gestures accompany the spoken words, while the third impact is inconsistent and contradictory):

- **Replication.** This is when the non-verbal behaviour echoes what is being said. The supervisor smiles and nods their head when saying, 'Well done, I am really glad you did that', or, with a slight shrug of the shoulders and open hands, says, 'Sorry, perhaps I got that wrong'.
- **Accentuation.** This is when non-verbal behaviour emphasizes aspects of the verbal message. The supervisor moves and leans more forward

demonstrating interest while saying, 'That is a very important point you raised; let's consider it in greater depth then'.

- **Inconsistency.** This is when there is a contradiction between the verbal and non-verbal messages. Consider these two examples:

  o The supervisee is saying they feel okay and that they will go ahead in making their request known to their manager, but their body language is telling you something different: you observe fidgeting and their voice is hesitant and more quiet than usual.

  o A supervisor says, 'Perhaps you need to be more open and honest in that situation', with arms tightly folded and legs crossed.

Perceiving non-verbal communication

By developing our conscious use of non-verbal cues and by recognizing the influence that non-verbal communication may have, we can begin to consider non-verbal messages from the supervisee. Watch for non-verbal cues while the other is speaking. What is their body language saying? Are their arms gesturing, or are they sitting back with arms folded? What are vocal patterns and gestures telling you that words can't? Are they speaking loudly, anxiously or quietly? Are their eyes wide open with excitement or looking tired from exhaustion? What does this suggest to you about how they feel about the topic they are discussing? Non-verbal communication can therefore raise our awareness and offer us clues to the underlying feelings or unexpressed thoughts of the supervisee. It is listening not only with our ears but with our eyes as well. Remember, though, that they are only clues, and how we interpret them may not be wholly accurate.

Heron (2001) describes six basic cues that we can pick up on that are evident in facial expressions and body language. I have chosen three, as we are taking our first steps, that a supervisor might perceive and make an effective response to:

- **Picking up on wanting to speak cues.** The supervisor is giving feedback and offering an alternative course of action. They pick up on the supervisee's facial expression and body movements that they want to say something. 'You look as if you want to stop me there, what do you need to say?'
- **Picking up on pensive cues.** The supervisee has a reflective and thoughtful look on their face; the supervisor asks an open question: 'What are you thinking?'
- **Picking up on emotion cues.** The supervisee has a look of surprise, delight, irritation, impatience or anxiety. The supervisor responds empathically: 'It looks as though you are . . .?', or by asking an open question: 'I'm wondering what you are feeling about that?'

Non-verbal communication is complex and multidimensional. We also need to be aware of cultural differences, norms and rules: the above examples may not always apply. The interested reader is directed to Morris (1994), Burgoon et al. (1996) and Lewis (2008), three books that consider the subject in detail, the latter two focusing on cultural differences.

There does need to be a balance in being yourself and being aware of your intentions and what the supervisee is wanting from you. Self-awareness is again important to be able to recognize what might be preoccupying you or making you appear anxious during the supervision. Is there something else on your mind or is it anxiety about saying or doing the right thing with your supervisee? The former you will need to find ways to leave behind, and the latter will be alleviated with practice and experience, although there always needs to be a certain level of anticipation and purposeful energy in your listening and responding. It is important, however, to be yourself, with your very own non-verbal manner, while remembering also to express your active listening and responding skills in the most effective way. Egan (2002) posits that it is your quality of being and presence with the person that is more important than non-verbal behaviour in itself. For a supervisor these are some of the values and the spirit that you bring to the sessions with your supervisee.

Reflective activity

Reflect on your non-verbal presence, using SOLER and the comments suggested here, in context to your supervision sessions, or when you have been in a similar role/situation.

- How effective are you in using postural cues to indicate your willingness to work with your supervisee?
- What are some ways you distract your supervisee from the task in hand?
- How natural are you with SOLER behaviours?
- What indicates to you that you are not being yourself?
- To what degree is your psychological presence (state of mind) reflected in your physical presence?
- What are you like when you are at your best?
- What are you like when you are at your worst?
- What do you have to do to become more effectively present to your supervisees both physically and psychologically?

Source: Adapted from Egan 2002

Remember that it is important to have self-awareness in being aware of our non-verbal communication. Remember also that it is not a case of getting these right or wrong – that can contribute to your feeling awkward and not yourself. Rather, it is being aware of what is more helpful and effective or less helpful and effective. As your self-assurance grows in supervising, learn to trust your intuition more. Stickley and Stacey (2009) point out that there are no universal guidelines when communicating non-verbally, and this applies equally to the supervision relationship.

Getting ready to listen

Effective listening requires the supervisor to be ready, both physically and mentally. Before your session starts, you will have prepared the room so it is free of distractions; now you need also to prepare yourself. Aim to take up to ten minutes before the session starts to collect your thoughts and to look at any notes from the previous meeting. You may need to remind yourself of certain details or of goals that were discussed. Your supervisee may have misremembered some of the detail since you last met and they will have other issues to talk about. It demonstrates your interest and care in them as a unique individual if you can recall relevant facts and information that has previously been discussed.

The next task is to get ready to listen. You may want to take a few minutes to relax and clear away any distracting thoughts and preoccupations that have nothing to do with the upcoming session. Think of them as internal interferences; you will inevitably be more focused if you can rid yourself of as many of them as you can.

The supervisor's toolbox of active listening skills

Use of questions

Asking questions might seem the most natural thing to do as a helper. This type of intervention is commonly used throughout daily tasks when you are gathering information and assessing needs. You will be carrying out these tasks in supervision. However, your role predominantly is to enable the supervisee to explore, while generally encouraging them to tackle and reflect on the issues that they are bringing to the session.

The types of questions that you ask are going to influence the kinds of responses you receive.

Closed questions

Closed questions can be answered with a short statement or fact, or more easily with a yes or a no. Examples are: 'How long have you worked there?', 'Do you often take charge of the ward?', 'Do you get much time to plan ahead?',

'Did you find that situation difficult?' Closed questions are of course necessary for your information gathering and to acquire facts. Often they are used at the beginning of sessions and when new issues are being introduced. However, they do not help in listening actively and are of limited use in helping the supervisor to reflect or to draw out the issues or concerns, as they do not facilitate exploration. Avoid overuse of closed questions as they can set up a question and answer pattern that may be hard to break.

Open questions

Open questions are more helpful for the supervisee as they leave the way open for a range of responses: they encourage a fuller picture. Closed questions can be made more open by asking:

- 'How do you feel when you take charge of the ward?'
- 'When are the best times for you to plan ahead?'
- 'What in particular did you find difficult when working with that patient?'

Although the asking of questions is not as straightforward as it seems, an open question can result in a limited answer as much as a closed question can bring about a longer response. What can influence this is the rapport you have with your supervisee. Rapport can be defined as an understanding and a connection that is developed in the relationship for the goal of supervision. It is important to keep this rapport in mind when supervising, although it will matter the most when you don't have it. However, as a general rule, ask open questions that help and enable the supervisee to explore, elaborate and focus on their experience and in reaching conclusions. Open questions can begin with how, what, when, where, who and why, although be cautious of the 'why' question and use it sparingly.

Why not use 'why' questions?

In therapeutic helping terms, and in particular when facilitating exploration, 'why' questions are best avoided, although there is some debate regarding their value (Sanders et al. 2009). 'Why' questions can be difficult to answer. Remember being asked as a child, 'Why did you do it?' 'Why' questions tend to make the person feel defensive, as they often sound judgemental, as though you expect the person to know the answer. The question can assume that we have a clear answer, but often it can invite an 'I don't know' response.

'Why' questions can make the supervisee feel pressured and then they may feel awkward or hurried into giving an unconsidered answer. Perhaps, above all else, avoid asking the 'why' question because the supervisee may not know why. I am not suggesting to avoid 'why' questions altogether: in certain contexts of helping they are useful. But be aware of their overuse and that alternatives, such as asking who, what, where, when and how, are more therapeutic, reflective, exploratory and supportive in their intention. Some examples of how 'why' questions might be changed are:

- 'Why did you do that?' becomes: 'I would like to understand your reasons behind that, what was going through your mind?', or 'When in particular does that occur?'
- 'Why did you say that to him?' becomes: 'What sort of response were you expecting?', or 'What were you expecting the outcome of that to be?'
- 'Why didn't you do what you said you would do?' becomes: 'I am wondering what happened that prevented you?'
- 'Why do you feel that way?' becomes: 'Who, in particular, were you feeling that with?', or 'When do you tend to have those feelings?'

Remember, too, before you ask a 'why' question, that the supervisee is possibly asking themself a similar 'why' question about the situation. What may benefit the most will be exploration and reflection, and not asking them why.

Using silence as a listening skill

It is important to recognize the value of silence in effective listening. However, in taking your first steps into supervision, silence as a listening skill may feel awkward and uncomfortable. Busy healthcare workers are more used to filling in all the gaps, getting things done as they are often in a rush. So silence perhaps does not come naturally in your repertoire of helping skills. I am not suggesting here long silences of the kind you may encounter when working with clients and patients, although the principles are similar. The focus here is on when there are pauses in the supervision dialogue, and how to use these for best effect. You may find at certain times in supervision that being silent is the most helpful expression that you can offer.

I remember when, as a new supervisor, I had a certain amount of nervousness. I was more focused on saying the right thing and appearing professional and competent than focusing fully on what the supervisee had to say. I did not want to give a wrong response. I would jump in too quickly with more questions. I was not giving enough space for the other person to think and reflect, and I was not fully appreciative of what silence could mean or how it could be used. Maybe there was an element of panic. However, with a little more experience and familiarity in the role I soon felt less anxious and was able to listen more. What also developed when I felt less pressured was that I became comfortable with silence and how to use silence therapeutically. I also learnt, as a listener, not to panic if there was silence.

When both you and your supervisee are taking the first steps in supervision, silence maybe awkward. You want to help out and immediately solve the problem. With increased confidence, understanding and insight of how silence can benefit, you can begin to use this skill to good effect.

It is important at first to ascertain when to allow silence to proceed or when it is better to break the silence with your dialogue. First to consider is which of you owns the silence. Is the supervisee being silent and taking time to reflect, or are you pausing to reflect? Consider also what the pause may signify. This may then help you regarding how to break the silence. Always ask yourself: Is my verbal intervention for their benefit and meeting their needs? Could this be valuable thinking and reflecting time before they explore further, or is the pause because they have come to a conclusion or exhausted the topic, and they are waiting for new direction? Am I breaking this silence because I am uncomfortable with it? If the last, then a helpful reflective moment will have been lost.

When to use silence

- At the start of a session, allowing time to settle, relax and focus attention on the session.
- When space is needed for thought and reflection.
- When space is needed for more exploration.
- When the supervisee needs to make a choice.
- When giving support non-verbally by communicating 'I am listening and here for you'.
- Just being there for the other person can indicate 'it's okay to be upset'.
- After giving feedback or making a challenge, allow reflective space.
- Silence should not be used as a substitute or excuse for not knowing how to respond. You could say, 'I am rather lost for words at the moment', or 'I need to think about that'.

Some responses to encourage or acknowledge the process of silence

- 'Spend a few moments, before we start, to collect yourself and your thoughts together.'
- 'I'm wondering what was going on for you then?'
- 'Take your time, you appear deep in thought.'
- 'You have said a lot there. [pause for a moment] Which issue you would like to discuss first?'
- 'You look a bit uncomfortable. I was wondering if you needed more time to think about that or if you were waiting for me to speak?'
- 'You don't need to respond straight away. Think about what I have just said.'

Silence and making good therapeutic use of the pause will further demonstrate your listening and empathic understanding to the other person. It also demonstrates that you are calm and relaxed, and communicates confidence in your supervisee, as you are allowing them to take responsibility for what are, at times, difficult decisions. Silences, when there is familiarity and understanding in the relationship, will usually become natural and spontaneous.

If you do feel you need to practise silence, a simple exercise is to pause for four or five seconds, when in conversation with someone, before you make your next response. This silence will become more natural and, as you gain more understanding of its meaning and use in supervision, can be used to good effect.

Reflecting and paraphrasing

Reflecting and paraphrasing are two skills that are used to feed back what the supervisee is saying, with the intention of communicating our understanding. However, they go much further than that. They also help the supervisee to explore the content further, to expand and develop thoughts and feelings with a view to gaining greater understanding. You may want to think of reflecting and paraphrasing as verbal rewards which give confidence and assurance to the supervisee that they can continue. Their experiences become more real by having verbalized them to you and can become explorative by your verbalizing them back. Both paraphrasing and reflecting encourage the supervisee to continue along their own route. View reflecting as a brief intervention that echoes back and highlights a crucial word or point that has just been spoken to you. Paraphrasing is a restatement, mainly your own words, that puts back to the other person the important thoughts and feelings that have been expressed to you. Reflecting and paraphrasing are also skills that communicate our empathic understanding and express our attitude of acceptance and respect towards the supervisee. These two skills are similar and in practice blend into each other. Together they are often referred to as reflective listening.

Reflecting

Reflecting back key words is the aural equivalent of holding up a mirror: the person gets to hear back what they are saying. It conveys your recognition of a key thought or feeling and confirms the presence of emotions. Along with that recognition you are adding weight to something important they have just said. If it was an emotion then reflecting can be a key to unlock further exploration. By reflecting back their words, or almost the exact words and perhaps idioms, then you are not judging or offering any opinion. The person begins to feel that what they have just said is valid and real. Reflecting back the particularly emotion-laden words begins to demonstrate your acceptance and empathy. For example:

Sue: I felt really upset when I found that out.
Supervisor: Upset?

Carl: It was all rather difficult; there were many mixed emotions.
Supervisor: Mixed emotions?

Both of these examples echo back key words and acknowledge what has been said. They help the supervisee to explore further and help clarify a key experience, e.g. what were the mixed emotions?

Carl: Yes, when we knew we had to break the news to him. Well, anyone would feel a bit stuck in knowing how to approach it.

Supervisor: You were feeling hesitant, perhaps a little nervous, and were not quite sure what you would say?

Here the supervisor is being empathic by sensing how Carl might be feeling, choosing a word and reflecting this back to him. The supervisor has also picked up that Carl is perhaps distancing himself, by not using 'I' statements and the real issue is still rather vague.

Carl: Yes, I guess I was. I was being tentative, even felt anxious and still don't know if I said the right thing or not.

The supervisor can now help Carl to focus in more detail. Carl felt safe to acknowledge his feelings and these can be further explored.

Think in terms of simple reflection and selective reflection. Simple reflection is when you echo back the same key word or short phrase such as 'You felt upset?' When being more selective you are reflecting back in your own words, in a tentative way, what they are not saying. As well as reflecting feeling, content can also be reflected.

Sue: All in all, I managed the situation to my best, by doing the right things.

Supervisor: It sounds as though you acted in a very professional way.

The supervisor could also have said 'You seem really pleased with yourself?', while also observing that Sue looks pleased and contented. Note that at the end of a reflective comment you are often employing an imaginary question mark: it is not a direct question you are asking but, by your intonation, you are inviting more.

Paraphrasing

Paraphrasing involves rephrasing, usually using fewer words, the essential meaning and context of a statement, or series of statements, that has just been said. You are attempting to get to the crux of the message, from the supervisee's frame of reference, and communicating first-level (basic) empathy. Remember being asked at school to read a piece of literature and then to 'put into your own words the following passages, to demonstrate that you have understood'. Paraphrasing can be thought of as similar, except that here it is alive and real with the intention of communicating so much more than just having a good memory. Restating the important and salient content not only continues and makes for a good relationship but also helps the supervisee to feel valued.

You can use paraphrasing most especially when there is a need for understanding during the conversations. You are testing and communicating your understanding without adding any new ideas to the other person's messages. A paraphrase demonstrates that you are listening and is aimed at being confirming and accepting. This enables the supervisee to further explore and express themselves. Usually a paraphrase needs to carry certain content if it is to be meaningful. Cameron (2008) emphasizes that paraphrasing has three components:

- Feelings
- Situations
- Behaviour

When paraphrasing, attempt to include two or more of these components: you are linking key issues for further reflection. They do not, however, need to be in any particular order. The following examples demonstrate this.

> Liz: It has been so busy and hectic lately, I have been rushing around all over the place. We are short staffed and I'm exhausted. I have simply had no time put in place some of the plans I have been discussing here.
> Supervisor: It seems that work [**situation**] is very demanding at the moment. You're getting worn out [**feelings**] and you have had no real time to develop those new procedures you wanted to [**behaviour**].

The paraphrase has an implied question that encourages the supervisee to further express their thoughts and feelings. I have inserted the three components of feelings, situation and behaviour in brackets. In the following examples look for these components yourself.

> Sam: To tell you the truth, I am really fed up at the moment and feel rather lost. My partner and I have just split up and I got a lousy appraisal last week. I feel like moving back to my home town.
> Supervisor: You feel disillusioned because you have had a relationship break up and a real setback at work. You are telling yourself to move back to somewhere that you know.

The response allows for more exploration as the supervisor avoids at first asking 'what happened?' or suggesting that the supervisee 'think twice about it'. The paraphrase gives a neutral focus.

In this next example the supervisor reflects back to expose and bring some clarity to mixed sentiments.

> Karim: It is generally going okay with the patient I spoke about last time, I think; most visits go really well but other times everything goes wrong. I don't understand why.
> Supervisor: Often you are pleased with the progress being made, but there is some puzzlement and concern for you, as some visits do not go the way

you would want and you're not fully grasping the reasons for that. What do you mean by everything goes wrong?

This allows for further exploration with a view to explore what Karim needs to do next or to change.

In a nursing context, the value of the paraphrase is not always appreciated, and Stein-Parbury (1993) notes that there is a reluctance to employ it. I have found this to be the case when training nurses in counselling skills: there is a reluctance at first to accept it in their repertoire of skills. Some do not recognize its value and so view it as pointless. Stein-Parbury says this reluctance stems from a fear of reinforcing the negative thoughts and feelings if they were to restate them back when a patient discloses their fears or anxieties. Perhaps also it is because nurses want to make things better for the patient and to be seen as having the answers when a worry or apprehension is expressed. I mention this here as it may help to acknowledge any awkwardness you may feel when beginning to use paraphrasing, and in doing so you can begin also to understand its purpose and to value it as a skill.

A word of warning

It is generally preferable to use you own words when paraphrasing, with the occasional key word(s) the supervisee has used. This avoids parroting, which can be annoying for your supervisee. Beware, too, the overuse of paraphrase as this becomes frustrating. Also, have an intention in mind as you paraphrase, otherwise the process of the conversation will just go round in circles. The other annoying facet can be when specific phrases such as 'what I hear you saying is', or 'so you are feeling' become constant in your repertoire. The repetitive use will begin to sound artificial and inauthentic. Stock phrases such as these, often used in training, you will hear yourself using, and to good effect. However, with further practice and skills in listening you will develop your own style, and paraphrasing can become a more natural form of communicating.

Clarifying

The skill of clarifying is important as clarifying is an opportunity to sort out any confusion in what the supervisee is saying. It is a means of checking understanding for both yourself and the other person. Clarifying can begin to expose some of the underlying issues that have been omitted from the narrative first time round and is a powerful way of focusing on important issues.

Clarification is also allied to being genuine in the relationship. You are being honest in admitting you are not clear about something or you would like to hear it again so you can more fully understand. This can enable the supervisee to double check and for them to be honest and admit to uncertainties. Clarifying can move a conversation forward, the important issues become more focused upon and the supervisee is clearer on what they really want to discuss.

Think of clarifying as having three aspects:

- **To check understanding**
  'It would help me understand better if you could give me an example of that?'
  'Where/when does that tend to happen?'
  'What, in particular, makes you respond in that way?'
  'Is that with any particular situation/person?'
  'Have I got that right, does it seem that way to you?'
- **To sort out confusion**
  'You seem to be saying two different things there. On the one hand you say you are happy at work yet you also say, with all the pressure at the moment you would leave tomorrow.'
  'I am a bit puzzled by what you have been describing. Pass it by me again with the effect it had on you.'
- **To focus on important aspects**
  'Which of those do you think we should focus on first?'
  'I am wondering what it is that really upset you with the incident you have just described.'

This type of questioning indicates your willingness to listen more as you may have missed something important. You are encouraging the supervisee to give more specific detail so you can both proceed further. Note the question mark at the end of a clarifying statement; your intonation will indicate that you are seeking greater clarification.

Self-disclosure

Self-disclosure is described here as an active listening skill: consider it as being a brief intervention with the intention of enabling the supervisee to further self-disclose and continue with their dialogue. The intention of self-disclosure is to create:

- Empathy
- Openness
- Risk taking
- Trust
- Further exploration

Through appropriate self-disclosure you can open up areas for further exploration, especially when you feel the supervisee is stuck or unsure about expressing themself more fully. Self-disclosure helps the supervisee to know that you are not afraid to be open and honest. Often we hold back from saying how we are feeling, there is a fear of being judged and embarrassed. We may consider it wrong or inappropriate that we feel in a particular way. Disclosing how you would feel in a similar situation lets the supervisee know it is okay. Indicating that such thoughts are not abnormal can be a very helpful experience.

By self-disclosing your own thoughts and feelings you are being open and honest, which can allow the supervisee to disclose and be more open. Empathy is shown by perceiving and recognizing some of their undisclosed thoughts. By taking a risk in disclosing how you would feel you are giving permission with an open invitation for the other person to take a risk.

Trust is developed as the supervisee gets to know you more closely, and self-disclosure helps to cement the bond. A sense of identification is gained by the supervisee and you are displaying equality in the relationship. The self-disclosure, however, needs to be genuine, sincere and congruent.

When self-disclosing be tentative and brief

Here are some examples of a supervisor's self-disclosure during their active listening with their supervisee:

- Beth has been talking rather anxiously about a meeting they are holding:

  Supervisor: I remember when I first had to chair a meeting, I was very nervous.

- Ben is reflecting on a situation when he had not being given the correct information. You pick up on his annoyance:

  Supervisor: I'm sure that if that had happened to me I would have felt angry.

- Simone is talking about being given some new responsibilities on top of her caseload and wondering how she might manage. She also appears to you to be rather worried:

  Supervisor: When I took on an extra role last year I found it difficult at first. I felt anxious about the new tasks I was being given and had some self doubt about whether I could perform them well. I am wondering if you are feeling something similar.

The objective and intention is to support the supervisee in feeling safe enough to self-disclose and explore some more.

Some guidelines when self-disclosing

- Keep it brief: the time is for the supervisee, not you.
- The supervisee's experience is the main focus; avoid taking attention away from the supervisee. Self-disclosure becomes unhelpful when the supervisee feels you have taken over the session.

- Avoid using phrases such as 'I know exactly what you are going through', or 'I know how you must be feeling', as they deny the supervisee's personal experience and individuality.

Summarizing

Summarizing is a skill that attempts to pull together broad themes and issues in what the supervisee has been discussing. Summarizing utilizes paraphrasing as it reflects back a number of statements and takes into acount the main feelings and thoughts that have been described. In this way it develops the process of empathy in the relationship. A good summary draws together the important points from the content and helps move the discussion forward. This enables the supervisee to get an overview and to see a fuller picture of what they have been discussing. It can help bring focus and clarity and assists in bringing direction and purpose to the session.

When to summarize

There is no golden rule, but you should certainly summarize near the end of the session. Leave enough time and opportunity for the supervisee to confirm the accuracy or put right any misunderstanding. To help with time boundaries you can announce that there are five minutes left and say 'Let us begin to summarize'. You will also want to include mini summaries from time to time. These help to focus and to keep on track, and are a reminder of what has been covered so far. Summaries are a good way of remembering. Be aware, however, that continual summarizing can become tedious.

Make a summary when an issue has been explored and you are now moving on to a different topic. When several issues have been brought to your attention, possibly at the beginning of a session, a summary is an invitation for the supervisee to choose which aspect to focus on first. For instance, 'You have mentioned several things there, you started by talking about [summarize] and then [summarize]; which would you like to focus on first?'

A summary is also useful when the supervisee is running off track or is getting stuck, for example, 'We seem to have reached a dead end there and are digressing; let's just pull together the main points and recap where you wanted to go with this.'

The more often you see your supervisee the more you will be able to make links in your summaries from previous sessions. For example, you can pick out themes from previous sessions to help identify areas to develop, or the salient points of their overall progress and achievements.

Learning to summarize

You will have many opportunities to practise summarizing in your everyday work setting. When listening to others, pick out and identify a key aspect of their dialogue in terms of experience, behaviour and the feelings experienced. A good summary will include the main aspect of each. Practise in appropriate situations by using those aspects to communicate the core message back to the speaker. Remember to check your accuracy; for example, 'Would that be a fair summary of what you have been saying so far?' You can also include a supportive statement or some positive feedback in a summary, to offer encouragement and motivation, such as, 'Knowing you as I do, you take on a new challenge with commitment and enthusiasm; I am sure what you have been saying is realistic to achieve.'

Remember, in a supervision context it will be a few weeks before you see the supervisee again, so end on a positive note whenever you can, as long as it is genuine and valid.

Conclusion

This chapter has focused on the necessary and essential skills of active listening and responding. With knowledge, awareness and possession of these skills you can proceed further in your development by integrating them into the full range of interventions that are possible in clinical supervision sessions. The next chapter will focus on categories of interventions, highlighting the skills, tasks and intentions each has for supervision.

Key learning points

- Understanding and defining the concept of active listening and responding skills will enable a supervisor to more readily focus on the task of supervising.
- A skilled supervisor recognizes and practises the key principles of active listening and responding.
- A therapeutic supervisor values active listening and responding by being empathic to the needs of the supervisee and to the tasks of supervision.
- A skilled supervisor recognizes the significance and importance of non-verbal communication.
- A skilled supervisor is able to use silence as a listening and responding skill.
- A skilled supervisor's toolbox contains a range of active listening and responding skills.

6

Six-category Intervention Analysis

Chapter outcomes

By reading this chapter, doing the reflective activities, and integrating the material into your supervision practice, you should be able to:

- Define the six categories of intervention analysis.
- Understand the importance and value of the six categories in relation to clinical supervision.
- Recognize and acknowledge distinct features and tasks of the six categories for clinical supervision.
- Know about and possess some skills of each of the six categories.
- Recognize and acknowledge degenerative interventions of the six categories.
- Recognize the importance of using the six categories for analysis and reflection.

Introduction

A model that is frequently offered as tool to both reflect and develop as a skilled helper is Heron's six-category intervention analysis (Heron 1975). This important framework is extremely useful to those who are new to supervision. It is indeed valuable to all supervisors who regularly reflect and review their therapeutic communication skills. When taking your first steps in supervision, this framework can be used for understanding and analysing the range of possible interventions you can make. Think of it as a practical tool whereby you can identify, monitor and review your skills and interactions with your supervisees.

Burnard (1985) and Burnard and Morrison (1988) introduced this as a framework to general nurse settings to develop skills, competence and effective helping in a broad range of interpersonal contexts. This conceptual model became influential in mental health nurse settings specifically in analysing the delivery of helping interventions for greater therapeutic value (Ashmore 1999; Morrissey 2009). It is a means of classifying varieties of effective communication between practitioners and clients. Indeed, it is equally applicable to any helping context where it is clear that helping is taking place and where the practitioner is offering an enabling service to the other person, as is the case with clinical supervision.

Although this is not a framework or model of clinical supervision, I and others (Bond and Holland 1998; Driscoll 2000; Sloan and Watson 2002), see six-category intervention analysis as a valuable learning context in which to develop supervision skills. As a framework it provides a therapeutic tool for supervisors to learn about, reflect on, monitor and develop interventions that are used during the sessions. It is also very much an attitude of mind which is rooted in humanistic psychology. It therefore provides a therapeutic base for the helping relationship. Heron (2001) uses the terms 'practitioner' and 'client', I have attempted to transfer that context to a supervision relationship, so 'supervisor' and 'supervisee' will mostly be used. The framework can become a powerful tool for personal and professional change. We can begin to recognize the six different styles and to identify which we use the most and the least frequently, and, most importantly, why? While none is better than the others, attention needs to be given to which are most appropriate for supervision and the service you are providing to your supervisee. As you become more familiar with the intentions of each of the categories, you will be able to develop a greater range of interventions within the six. This will then enable you to select the more appropriate and therapeutic intervention that meets the needs of the supervisee.

The value of six-category intervention analysis to the clinical supervisor

The value of intervention analysis to the clinical supervisor may be summarized as follows:

- It identifies a wide range of possible interventions that are available to the clinical supervisor.

- By identifying and applying a range of interventions the supervisor can act more precisely and supervise with a greater sense of intention and flexibility.
- It enables the supervisor to become aware of alternatives to their more normal style in practice.
- The analysis offers a means for training along with personal and professional development for the role of clinical supervisor.
- It enables the supervisor to become aware of strengths and weaknesses in each of the categories.
- It encourages analysis of how different interventions elicit different responses.
- Effective and therapeutic interventions used will enable the supervisee to reflect and problem solve, while feeling valued and supported.
- Effective and therapeutic interventions will more likely enable the supervisee to develop as a practitioner and use supervision more productively.

The word 'intervention' is used to describe any verbal or non-verbal behaviour that the supervisor may use as part of the interaction with the supervisee. There are six categories of helping styles but there are numerous interventions that can fall within the six. Heron (2001) claims that the six categories comprehend all desirable and worthwhile types of intervention. The framework is shown in Figure 6.1.

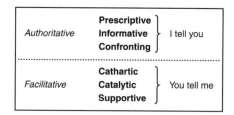

FIGURE 6.1 Heron's six-category intervention analysis

The first three categories are called **authoritative**; in each case the supervisor is taking a more overtly dominant role. The supervisor is taking responsibility for directing the conversation and is more in control by asking or telling the supervisee. The emphasis in the definition is on what the supervisor is doing: the 'I am telling you' in Figure 6.1. The second set of three are called **facilitative** since the role of the supervisor is less obtrusive and more discreet. The supervisor is less in control, seeking to enable the supervisee to take more responsibility and asking the supervisee to tell. The emphasis in the definition is on the effect of the intervention on the supervisee: 'You tell me' in Figure 6.1.

The value or intention of each category is demonstrated in Figure 6.2 with examples of the type of intervention used by a supervisor during a supervision session.

Category	Value of the intervention
1. Prescriptive	The supervisor directs and guides the supervisee, for example by giving advice or suggestions, to increase and develop self-determination
2. Informative	The supervisor provides information to impart new knowledge to the supervisee, for example by instructing, explaining or by giving examples from practice or experience
3. Confronting	The supervisor challenges the supervisee's thinking, beliefs, behaviour, values or attitudes, for example by offering and giving feedback or sharing a hunch of what you think is holding them back. This does not imply confrontation. The supervisor is seeking to raise the supervisee's awareness and help them to avoid making the same mistakes again
4. Cathartic	The supervisor helps the supervisee to express their feelings and fears, for example by communicating empathic understanding and facilitating the release of pent-up or unexpressed feelings
5. Catalytic	The supervisor seeks to enable the supervisee to learn, reflect, generate new options and problem solve, and so to become increasingly more self-directive, for example by active listening and responding and then actively listening some more
6. Supportive	The supervisor seeks to reinforce the confidence and affirm the worth and value of the supervisee, for example by demonstrating and communicating care, concern, enthusiasm and respect

FIGURE 6.2 Six-category intervention analysis applied to clinical supervision

There is no implication that any category is either more or less significant than any other. They are not distinguished by differences in value or merit. In principle, in relation to each other, one is no more positive or negative. The importance is determined by the nature of the intervention and the response of the supervisor to the needs of the supervisee or supervision. You will find that each has a high value in the appropriate context depending on the situation and the supervisor's role. Bearing this in mind, a skilful and self-aware supervisor aims for the following:

- To be equally proficient in all six categories, with a wide range of interventions in each one.
- To know when to be direct and to lead the supervisee (authoritative) and when to follow by facilitation.
- To be able to move elegantly and skilfully from one type of intervention to another as the developing situation and purpose of the interaction require.
- To be aware that the value of the intervention is in the context of their role and function as a supervisor.

I now offer an overview of each of the categories, including relevant interventions that would be applicable for the supervisor. Alongside developing awareness of valid and therapeutic interventions, Heron (2001) highlights the negative interventions that are possible in the six categories. He classifies one form of non-therapeutic interventions as degenerative. I will refer to these as pitfalls that a supervisor can slip into. The following categories identified are from Heron (2001); I have adapted the material in each to a clinical supervision context, unless stated otherwise.

The prescriptive category

The intention of this category is to direct or influence the supervisee's behaviour and actions in relation to their role as a healthcare worker. The aim is to prescribe ways of thinking and goals for behaviour. This is distinct from prescribing behaviour itself, unless it is to be on moral, ethical or legal grounds. The objective is for the supervisee to act with greater self-determination in purposeful co-operation with others.

Ways in which the supervisor can be prescriptive

- Making suggestions
- Making requests
- Proposing
- Giving advice
- Persuading
- Commanding

I have arranged the list in the order shown to demonstrate that the prescriptive interventions can range from soft direction, making suggestions, to hard direction, making commands. For prescriptive interventions to be valid and therapeutic, they should be made in the true interest of the other person. Prescriptive interventions, when used appropriately, can help bring about major insight or new understanding for the supervisee.

When a prescriptive intervention is appropriate

A general rule to bear in mind is that prescriptive interventions are best offered when the focus is on technical or practical matters. It is not recommended, or so easy, to give advice on matters regarding relationships, feelings or on aspects of how the other person should live their life. You may want to offer facts, but not opinions.

There are circumstances when a prescriptive intervention is appropriate:

- If there is a crisis which needs rapid action.
- The subject or issue discussed is genuinely incomprehensible to the supervisee and they need more expert guidance.
- There are right or wrong answers to questions or issues raised, for example concerning policies, procedures, legal aspects or ethical issues.
- You need to encourage the supervisee to check the facts with other experts.
- The supervisee, for whatever reason, is not in a position to make their own decision.

Some examples of giving direction

If the supervisee is in severe difficulties then giving prescriptions can be a caring and responsible form of both helping and protecting them:

- 'I feel you really need to speak to your manager about that and as soon as possible.'

When you feel or know there is a breach of a rule or regulation then you need to give advice in a strong and firm manner:

- 'I strongly recommend this ... course of action otherwise ... that will happen.'
- 'It is essential that you do that as soon as possible, otherwise ... will be the consequence.'

Bond and Holland (1998) point out that when giving strong advice it is preferable to be positive, using do's rather than don'ts in the language. For example, 'Don't use confusing jargon next time you speak with him', is better expressed as 'Do make that clear with the patient.'

It could be argued that one aim of supervision is to develop the effectiveness of the supervisee by drawing out their own reflections and resourcefulness while focusing on their healthcare practice. The more you let go of wanting to give your advice and opinions the more you will be able to achieve that. It would then follow that if we genuinely have faith in the supervisee then we would hold back from being prescriptive. Being too ready and eager to give advice may indicate that you have no faith in the process of clinical supervision. Also be aware of when you may be rescuing the supervisee by giving advice. Their discomfort at a puzzling situation may be in fact your discomfort, either of not knowing the answer or of having to sit through the session with their anxiety in front of you (Bond and Holland 1998).

Some examples of soft directions

- 'Would you like me to give you some advice on that matter?'
- 'This is only my opinion ...'

- 'An option that springs to my mind is . . .'
- 'You could possibly think about it this way . . .'
- 'What do you think about the suggestion I have just put to you?'

Holding back on giving advice

A new and inexperienced supervisee may come to supervision expecting advice and direction. There may be times when they will ask for advice outright before any exploration or thought.

Some examples of holding back on giving advice when asked are:

- 'Well, I could give you my opinion, but I am sure you will profit more by considering what you think first?'
- 'I wish I could tell you, but I feel you really need to mull over that for yourself. Let's explore it some more.'
- 'So, if you were me, what would you do?'
- 'Just imagine you could see the way forward with that. What would it look like?'
- 'Let us first consider all the options and then rate them all for positives and negatives.'
- 'You could do some reading around that subject and we can share some ideas next time we meet.'

Those are just some ways you can put the request for advice back to the supervisee, and I am sure you will find your own variations. The aim is to help and enable the supervisee to develop their own thoughts and ideas, while still engaging in the process and being supportive yourself. Of course, if they are completely stuck then hard direction is needed.

Some degenerative outcomes and pitfalls of prescriptive interventions

- It is open to the supervisor's taking over the problem of the supervisee.
- Overriding the supervisee's autonomy and responsibility by giving advice when it is not needed.
- Supervisees can become demoralized at all you know about them which they don't understand themselves.
- Can create a dependent supervisee.
- Not being assertive in giving advice; by being hesitant and indecisive when a strong course of action is called for.
- Large-scale interpretations can easily be used to demonstrate the skills and knowledge of the supervisor at the expense of the supervisee's working things out for themself.
- A need to show and impress the supervisee with all that you know.

(Adapted from Heron 2001)

The informative category

The intention of this category is to give new knowledge, information or meaning in relation to the supervisee's role as a healthcare worker. The aim is to give information which the supervisee sees as relevant and of interest and thereby to encourage the supervisee to be an active partner in the learning process. The overall objective is to enable the supervisee to make informed judgements and decisions, and to think rationally when taking action. Informative interventions serve to move the supervisee forward to a new understanding and can offer the supervisee a more immediate interpretation of the current situation. They are less authoritative than prescriptive interventions; Bond and Holland (1998) distinguish between these categories stating that giving information is sharing facts, opinions and procedures whereas giving advice is offering examples of specific courses of action.

Ways in which the supervisor can give information

- Offering new facts and information
- Sharing knowledge and opinions
- Teaching
- Self-disclosing
- Interpreting
- Instructing
- Refer to alternative sources

When information giving may be appropriate

- The situation is urgent and needs rapid action.
- The supervisee is stuck in their thinking.
- The supervisee is stuck in a cycle of behaviour which is becoming unhelpful or even destructive.
- A gap in knowledge or misunderstanding is contributing to the problem that they are experiencing at the present time.
- Clarification is needed on certain key points or facts that they are bringing to your attention.
- The supervisee has decided on a course of action which may have inappropriate consequences; information or advice is needed to reconsider.
- When the supervisee's confidence is low, and offering important information or advice can help to overcome their difficulties.

(Adapted from Bond and Holland 1998)

Some principles of information giving

- Identify what the supervisee wants to know.

- Clarify what they already understand about the subject.
- Assess the accuracy of their current knowledge.
- Use understandable and appropriate language.
- Be clear and specific.
- Clarify the supervisee's comprehension and understanding.
- Discuss others' reaction to information.
- Back up with written information and evidenced-based practice.

(Adapted from Stein-Parbury 1993)

Some examples of giving information

- 'What is your understanding of that procedure?'
- 'What experience have you had dealing with that kind of incident?'
- 'Would you like some information on that? What in particular do you want to know?'
- 'I feel I need to correct you there, check the policy again; there is a copy in the office.'
- 'There is a specialist who may be able to help, I can give you contact details.'
- 'When something similar happened to me I found it helpful to . . .'
- 'These are my thoughts on the subject.'
- 'So, feed back to me what you have learnt from that.'
- 'What are some of your thoughts on that theory?'
- 'Check that out with others as well.'

As a general rule, bring information giving into the flow of the session and keep it brief: you want to avoid a long dialogue that turns into a teaching session. Try to use open questions to start with, as in the first two examples above. If the giving of information is used well, the supervisee becomes an active partner in the learning process.

Some degenerative outcomes and pitfalls of informative interventions

- Too frequent information giving can remove important learning from the supervisee.
- Can create a dependent supervisee.
- Giving an abundance of information that is not relevant to their situation can overwhelm and confuse the supervisee.
- Be aware of tone of voice and body language when giving information. Looking surprised by their lack of knowing can be a put-down and make the supervisee feel stupid.
- If you make a promise regarding information gathering, make sure you do deliver and bring the information into the next session.
- The temptation to appear the wise leader (guru) has to be recognized.

(Adapted from Heron 2001)

The confronting category

The intention of this category is to raise awareness about some limited attitude or behaviour which the supervisee is relatively unaware of. The aim is to develop and create insight for the supervisee for personal and professional growth. Confronting interventions involve challenging aspects of the supervisee's behaviour that are restrictive and giving of constructive feedback.

Cutcliffe and Epling (1997) support the use of appropriate and skilful challenging in clinical supervision for the personal and professional development of the supervisee. Faugier (1992) also advocates growth and development occurring in supervision. So it is important here to consider principles and skills of effective challenging. There is also a section on challenging skills in Chapter 7 and the appropriate use in a model of problem solving.

The supervisor's reluctance to challenge

The skill of challenging, which is often referred to as the art of challenging, can be a difficult area for the new supervisor to grasp. Indeed, many supervisors remain reluctant to challenge their supervisee and have ways of avoiding having to do so. Some common self-defeating statements and justifications that allude to this reluctance are:

- 'Challenging is contrary to my style of healthcare, I am not used to doing it that way.'
- 'I do not want to hurt my supervisee's feelings.'
- 'I have misgivings about challenging, based on past experiences.'
- 'I will challenge them if it happens again; someone else might point it out to them in the meantime.'
- 'I need to get to know the supervisee first; it is far too early in the relationship to challenge.'
- 'My supervisee needs support rather than to be challenged.'
- 'If I was to challenge my supervisee they may get angry or upset and not want to come back.'
- 'They may no longer like or respect me.'
- 'I like being nice.'

Tips and techniques for challenging the supervisee

A reluctance to challenge may be due to minimal or no constructive training in the effective use of challenging skills. Research studies by Morrison and Burnard (1998) indicate that nurses use the confronting category the least of the six as it was discomforting to use and not generally in the nature of their work. It would seem logical to suggest that nurses who are becoming clinical supervisors may also hesitate, feel uncertain about, or lack skills in, challenging. The danger here is that with the reluctance to challenge there is going to be avoidance. Confronting and challenging should not be confused with confrontation. To challenge the supervisee in the spirit of supervision, certain principles and techniques need to be in place.

- Build a relationship that has a balance of support and challenge.
- Be empathic.
- Be tactful and tentative.
- Use an 'I' message, not 'you' message, when beginning to challenge. For example, 'I notice there are quite a few negative thoughts about that person', rather than 'You are being very negative describing that relationship'. The latter can put the supervisee on the defensive whereas the former is more neutral and an invitation to explore.
- Present your own alternative and perspective.
- Share factual information.
- Share your hunches.
- Help the supervisee to explore alternative perspectives.
- Invite the supervisee to challenge themself.
- Challenge strengths rather than a weakness.
- Allow the supervisee the opportunity to respond.
- Summarize the central issues and seek clarification of learning and understanding.

Challenging well is an art, and is developed through practice. Challenging skills are strong medicine (Egan 2002): they can have strong healing and relieving effects but they can also have side effects if not administered correctly or if no warning is offered. Often I hear training supervisors say they need to build up the relationship first to a safe level and they need to get to know the supervisee before challenging. I tend to disagree with that viewpoint. You need to dip your toe in the water from the start, and I believe it is better to start as you mean to go on and have challenging as an open and honest part of your working style from the beginning and not as something you suddenly bring into the sessions a few months down the line. This can have the effect of startling the supervisee; they wonder what they have suddenly done wrong or differently. It may increase their anxiety as they ask themself, 'Why is my supervisor suddenly challenging me now?' But remember from the outset that the amount of challenge certainly needs to be balanced with support.

Examples of challenging

There are dangers involved in making a challenge: you may not know the best words to use, whether the timing is right or how the supervisee may respond to you. However, you can pre-empt some of these dangers by announcing a challenge in a tentative way. Here are two examples:

- 'Would it feel okay if I was to challenge you on that, as I have just noticed something you said?' [and then wait for the response]
- 'It feels rather risky to say this to you and I really hope I am not putting our relationship in jeopardy, but I am going to challenge you on that thought.' [then make the challenge]

Use supportive interventions with the challenge, for example:

- 'I feel you have the insight and strength to take this on board, so I am going to give you some feedback which might help.'

If you take challenge into the general conversation the supervisee will be accustomed to your style of working from the word go; it also enables the learning and development to stay alive and creative.

Some degenerative outcomes and pitfalls of confronting interventions

- Talking around the issue because of your anxiety about raising it.
- Apologizing profusely and insisting that the supervisee does not feel too bad about you for having to say this. This has the effect of giving away the responsibility you have in this important function of being a supervisor.
- The sledgehammer approach, a term used by Heron (2001) to describe the situation when the issue is raised aggressively, with no tact or sensitivity, so it becomes an attack.
- Being authoritarian, telling the supervisee off as though they were a naughty child.

(Adapted from Heron 2001)

Confronting interventions should not be confused with confrontation as the intention is very different. Heron (2001) refers to challenging as offering a gift with the capacity to enhance understanding and insight rather than highlighting negative aspects of an individual.

It also needs to be noted that confronting interventions differ from the others in that they are generally not asked for and often not expected. The supervisor is presuming to judge what the other is unaware of and therefore presuming the intervention will be in their interest. As a supervisor, you are in a unique and privileged position: you have permission to offer challenge and feedback, as this was part of the learning and working agreement. Such a privilege only serves to highlight that this category needs to be delivered with skill and composure.

Reflective activity

Recall several situations, in your role as a healthcare worker, when you have been challenged by somebody on an aspect of your work.

Think back to one of those situations where you felt it was negative and left you feeling worse or confused. Make notes on the following:

- What did the person do and say?
- How was the challenge delivered?
- How were you left feeling?

Now think back to a situation when you were challenged in a positive way, one where you gained insight which enabled you to make some positive changes, and where you felt supported. Make notes on the following:

- What did the person say and do?
- How was it delivered?
- How were you left feeling?

Now ask yourself:

- What can you learn from these two experiences?
- What did the person in the second situation do that the other did not?
- How will your own experiences of being challenged be helpful to you as a supervisor?
- Being honest with yourself, what do you feel you need to be challenged on during supervision?
- How would you want this to be delivered to you?
- Would you ever ask to be challenged on an aspect of your work or role?
- Are there any discrepancies in how you are going to use challenge as a supervisor and how you would want to be challenged as a supervisee?
- What do you feel you need to work on and develop with your own challenging skills?
- How will you achieve this?

From the above activity you have probably gained some insight into what makes a positive challenge and a negative one. Also, the intention was for you to challenge yourself to develop this category of intervention for appropriate use in clinical supervision

The cathartic category

The intention of cathartic interventions is to enable the supervisee to release pent-up and repressed emotions. The aim is for the supervisee to have expression and control in developing emotional competence by being be more open and aware of feelings and having greater understanding of them.

Rungapadiachy (1999) rightly points out that cathartic intervention should not be taken lightly. In managing emotional release from the supervisee you need to feel confident, comfortable and skilled. It is likely that you will meet with the feelings of the supervisee as they talk about their frustrations, concerns, hopes, sadness and the many other emotions that occur in their practice as a helper. It is also of value to remember that the intention in the cathartic category is the release of feelings, rather than the talking about them. For whatever reason, emotions may not be expressed, and it is not your task to make that happen. Heron (2001) states that there needs to be an agreement in the helping relationship, meaning that any intention to be cathartic should occur only with permission. In supervision there is an agreed contract to work together. However; this does not include personal therapy, so we need to be cautious here. Catharsis may possibly take place voluntarily, without any intent on your part, so you do need to be ready and able to help the supervisee. With respect to skills, at the very least you will need to be able to contain feelings and emotions, if they emerge, with confidence, competence and understanding.

Some examples of cathartic interventions

- 'You seem very angry, that's okay, and let it out if you want.'
- 'Take your time.' [pause and use silence to demonstrate non-verbal listening]
- 'You look upset and even a bit tearful talking about what happened.'
- 'Would it help to explore how you feel a bit more deeply?'
- 'That situation appears to have really got to you. What do you need right now?'
- 'What would you really like to say to him?'

These are examples of cathartic interventions when your intention is to help the supervisee express, release and discharge feelings and emotion, when you feel it is appropriate and in their best interest to do so. They are stated with a sense of asking permission and a genuine affirmation that it is okay to do so.

Some degenerative outcomes and pitfalls of cathartic interventions

Probably the most common pitfalls are interventions that block catharsis or turn the attention away from the emotion when there would be therapeutic benefit in expressing that emotion. For example:

- 'I am sure it will be just fine, you just wait and see.'
- 'No point dwelling on it, it's done, let's move on.'

Although your intention is to be supportive, you are ignoring or avoiding the feelings associated with the issue being raised. This avoidance can possibly be because you are uncomfortable with the feelings or unsure how to handle them. Your supervisee may pick up on this and thus avoid disclosing, as they feel you would be unable to contain the emotions.

Some other pitfalls are:

- Not recognizing, or avoiding, body cues and non-verbal behaviour that quite possibly indicate the supervisee is angry, upset, frustrated, etc.
- Analysing and interpreting the feelings on behalf of the supervisee without qualification. For example, you assume that they are dissatisfied and you make a point of letting them know why and how.
- By being unskilled and lacking in competence and the consequences of catharsis could be muddled as you both reach for the tissues and need support.

The catalytic category

The intention of catalytic interventions is to encourage supervisee problem solving, reflection, self-discovery and learning within the context of the supervision relationship and also beyond it. The aim will be for development in self-awareness, understanding and insight.

Catalytic interventions are central to personal development work with other people (Heron 2001). They are therefore central in developing the supervision relationship, which is built on the three core conditions, and the subsequent work that is to take place. Consider catalytic skills to be essential for facilitating the topics and thoughts that the supervisee brings to the sessions. A catalyst can be defined as someone or something that helps to bring about change without itself interfering or becoming part of it. As supervisor you are therefore providing both the space and the vehicle for exploration, development and change to occur.

Key skills

- Open questions
- Prompts and probes
- Reflecting
- Paraphrasing
- Clarifying
- Self-disclosure (discreet and appropriate)
- Summarizing

These key skills form the foundations of all types of supervision interventions and have already been explored in Chapter 5. In Heron's six-category framework they are classified and recognized as a distinct category to enable you in your own analysis and development of skills.

Some degenerative outcomes and pitfalls of catalytic interventions

- Too many closed questions can rush the supervisee into wrong answers and also narrow the field of opportunity to explore further.
- As supervisor you seek order to the discussion because of your own need to search for a meaning and reach a solution, and as quickly as possible. Your seemingly open questions can be disguised as a prescribing intervention: for example, 'Don't you think it would be a good idea if . . .?, or 'Stop there, have you not thought about . . .?'
- The above examples can also be when you want to close and reach a tidy ending to meet your own need for completion on that particular issue.
- Drawing out information and material that is going to satisfy your own curiosity or need to hear gossip. As catalytic interventions are means of prompting and probing, and are thus potentially powerful skills, they can be manipulated to encourage the supervisee to overdisclose: for example, 'Tell me some more of what you overheard?'
- Answering your own questions. For example, 'How do you think she felt at that point? She was sure to be angry?' These are known as leading questions because they indicate the answer you expect.
- Using catalytic skills in a compulsive way, where you keep reflecting back and paraphrasing and end up going around in circles rather than giving advice or information when the supervisee is stuck or asking for clarification.
- Being distracted by your own material so you are not focusing in the here and now with your supervisee and not actively listening.

(Adapted from Heron 2001)

The supportive category

The intention of supportive interventions is to affirm the worth and value of the supervisee as a person and in their role as a healthcare worker. The aim is to provide therapeutic care and support for the supervisee in order that they might develop a more positive self-image personally and professionally. Bringing the supervisee to a fuller appreciation of themselves is an essential element of supervision. If that is to take place it is very likely that your supervisee will have more appreciation of others as well.

Supportive interventions can be viewed and analysed as distinct and separate from the other categories, but they also need to run deep in all interventions. Heron (2001) calls for the helper to have an attitude of mind of being supportive, that underpins all the categories of intervention. Bond and Holland (1998: 133) also state that the clinical supervisor *'needs to be fundamentally supportive at all times'*.

Essential qualities and values

The supervisor is:

- Nurturing
- Accepting
- Affirming
- Genuine
- Warm
- Empathic
- Respectful

The supervisor has the values to:

- Be supportive to the supervisee as a person.
- Be supportive of the supervisee's qualities.
- Be supportive of their beliefs and values.
- Be supportive of their actions and behaviour (that fall within ethical and moral boundaries and codes of conduct).
- Be supportive of their creations and projects in other aspects of their life.

Some supportive skills and interventions

- In the general scheme of things, supervision time is short, so give support often and explicitly.
- Give a warm welcome and greeting at the beginning of the session.
- Use of the supervisee's name and refer to them by name often.
- Express positive feelings.
- Express care and concern: for example, 'I do care what happens', or 'I do hope that will turn out well for you', and 'my concern for you about that is . . .'
- Give encouragement by pointing out the supervisee's achievements and strengths and urge the supervisee to voice these.
- Be their advocate and verbally back them up during the session, for example when they deserve better support, recognition or respect from others.
- Apologize for your mistakes, without making lame excuses, and for any lack of consideration, as this communicates respect.
- Verbally celebrate successes and encourage the supervisee to acknowledge these as well.

- Give free attention, for example staying silent with genuine intent when the supervisee is reflecting internally.
- Use appropriate self-disclosure by sharing your own experiences and feeling with the intention of being supportive.

Some degenerative outcomes and pitfalls of supportive interventions

- Giving qualified support: for example, 'You are very conscientious but it is a shame that you . . .'
- Overdone support; when your praise becomes excessive it can sound false.
- Patronizing. Be aware of talking down to your supervisee as a parent would to a child, for example when calm is needed. Although no ill may be intended, I feel the short phrase 'oh bless' may be perceived as patronizing. However genuine the intent, it can possibly have connotations such as trying to be kind, nice or not knowing what else to say. To some it may sound like sympathy in disguise, for example 'you poor thing', or even a veiled criticism, 'stupid idiot'.
- Not recognizing when support is needed, for example not picking up on anxious or awkward body language when the supervisee really needs you to say something.
- Lack of appropriate non-verbal response, for example not smiling when the supervisee is pleased with themselves.
- Showering the supervisee with help and taking on too much responsibility when they are upset or going through a difficult time. This is often known as rescuing and is probably meeting your own needs while having the effect of negating the supervisee's own resources.

(Adapted from Heron 2001)

Six-category intervention analysis for clinical supervision

The six categories are not totally exclusive of each other. They can and do integrate by being significantly and necessarily interdependent. For example:

- When giving advice you back this up with information: for example 'I suggest you read up on that subject to update yourself [prescriptive] the library here will assist you with a literature search [informative].'
- When challenging your supervisee you also offer support: 'You usually do take time out when you can, and help students who you see struggling [supportive] but while talking about this one, I notice you raise your voice and appear rather irritated, would I be right in saying that? [challenge]'

Remember also non-verbal interventions, for example following an open question as an invitation to talk [catalytic] on a matter of real concern, you use non-verbal communication and gestures of support and warmth.

However, the six categories of intervention have relatively pure forms and are and can be clearly distinguished from each other. In order to develop analysis and recognition of the categories think about what your intention is and the purpose you want it to serve the supervisee. It is the intention of the intervention that distinguishes one from another. With each individual intervention you make, the general purpose or thrust should be clear and be integral to the needs of the supervisee.

It is important to remember that the **authoritative interventions** generally need to be delivered with a **facilitative** intent. For example, you are:

- Helping your supervisee to be more autonomous and responsible regarding their actions [**prescriptive**].
- Enabling understanding and learning [**informative**].
- Raising self-awareness [**confronting**].

Conversely, the **facilitative interventions** need to be delivered with a certain amount of **authority** in the sense that you do know what you are doing and why. For example, you:

- Have a strong and genuine commitment to be **supportive**.
- Have the skills, knowledge and experience to facilitate by prompting and probing, reflecting, problem solving and exploring [**cathartic** and **catalytic**]. Heron (2001) proposes that for all categories to have a therapeutic impact they need the desired catalytic input and a foundation of support. For example, when prescribing or informing, ask open questions first for the supervisee's thoughts or understanding. When giving constructive feedback by confronting there need to be supportive statements by giving positive comments and affirming the person's worth and value.

Key points about valid and degenerative interventions

Valid interventions are appropriate to the situation, the supervision relationship and the agreement. This means that the intervention is:

- In the right category.
- The right type of intervention within the category.
- Right in content, and use of language is appropriate.
- Delivered in the right manner.
- Delivered with good timing.

When you are reflecting back on the session with a view to assessing what might be more therapeutic in the future, use this simple framework and ask yourself:

- Was it the correct category for what was going on in the interaction with the supervisee?
- If the category was right, was it the right intervention within the category?

If so, was:

- The content appropriate?
- The manner appropriate?
- The timing good?

Degenerative interventions fail in one, and usually several, of above aspects because of the supervisor's lack of experience or awareness. Degenerative interventions are misguided rather than intentional.

Reflective activity

Note: When in doubt about recognizing a category you are to use, ask yourself: What is my intention? For example, is my intention to be prescriptive or informative?

Now ask yourself:

- Within your work setting and role as a healthcare worker, which of the six categories do you use most of?
- Least of?
- Is this due to the type of work you carry out or to a lack of skill and experience?

Thinking now about your supervision ask yourself:

- Which of the interventions may you possibly overuse?
- Which of the interventions may you possibly underuse?
- How will you recognize when an intervention is valid and therapeutic?
- How will you recognize when an intervention is less appropriate, misguided and therefore degenerative?
- What factors may enhance and hinder your application of certain interventions with your supervisee?
- Which of the six categories do you need to develop for your supervision practice?
- What interventions within that category do you need to develop?
- How will you achieve this?
- How will you know when you have?

Further use of the six categories for your supervisee

The more you gain knowledge and understanding of this framework of helping interventions the more you will be able to recognize your supervisee's range of skills they use as a helper in their work setting. When your supervisee reflects on issues from practice, you can develop their self-awareness by helping them to evaluate and reflect on the effectiveness of their interventions. You can give feedback both positive and constructive regarding the valid and not so valid interventions they have used. Ask what the intention was, for example, when a particular interaction with a client had not been helpful. Help them explore other possible styles of communication that might have been more appropriate. You may have a supervisee who avoids challenging or who gets it all wrong when they do. You may want to help them explore their range of challenging skills and some pitfalls they find themselves slipping into. You can pass on your experience and skills by becoming, and being, a good role model with this type of intervention. You will be able to help your supervisee to develop and evaluate their own range of interventions, so they can become more effective and therapeutic in their healthcare role.

Reflective activity

With your understanding of six-category intervention analysis, can you think of other ways you can transfer this knowledge to enable your supervisees to develop their range of communication skills in their own healthcare setting?

The need to be aware of degenerative interventions

I feel it is important to provide a brief sketch of the degenerative interventions as these are often *'misguided, rooted in lack of awareness, lack of experience, of insight, of personal growth or simply of training'* (Heron 2001: 186).

There are at least four kinds of degenerative intervention (Heron 2001).

1 **Unsolicited.** When a practitioner appoints themself in the role of helper, and without being asked starts to give advice, instructs, confronts or finds other ways to help that are disrespectful and interfering to the other person's autonomy.

In supervision, a form of this may manifest when the supervisor intervenes and tells the supervisee what to do and how to do it before establishing if that is what they want. There needs to be a principle of respect for personal autonomy and responsibility, even after allowing for the freely chosen contract, such interventions require a preface such as, 'Can I offer you some advice on that?'

2 **Manipulative**. Practitioners are motivated by their own self-interest regardless of the interests of the client; the focus is on them rather than the client. Motives are for self-gratification and satisfaction.

In supervision, a form of this may manifest when the supervisor becomes nosy and steers the supervisee to talk about certain personal matters, or to find out the gossip that is happening on the ward.

3 **Compulsive**. The practitioner has unresolved and unacknowledged personal problems that interfere with therapeutic helping. Emotional competence in dealing with a variety of helping situations in different ways has not been developed. Some traits of compulsive helpers can be seen as always working too hard, taking on too much responsibility, wanting to be liked or always wanting to take control. That is not to say that there is no time or place for such activities. It is when that type of helping is done over and over again at the expense of more desirable interventions that it becomes a problem. The practitioner only has available a small number of the six types of intervention, so there is a limited range, and they are frequently misapplied.

In supervision, a form of this may manifest in the supervisor's always wanting to be nice, to pamper, look after at all costs, mollycoddle and collude with the supervisee, when challenging may have been more appropriate. Or the supervisor always wants to solve the problem as soon as it is being told.

4 **Unskilled**. The practitioner has a limited repertoire of skills or is incompetent for the required therapeutic activity or interaction. Interventions are ad hoc and variable with respect to quality and suitability.

In supervision, a form of this will manifest when the supervisor has had no formal training and lacks experience or transferable skills for clinical supervision. There can be numerous occasions when the supervisor will be out of their depth and offer unskilled interventions. For example:

Supervisee: I think I gave some wrong information about some possible side effects of the medication he was asking about. I got a bit mixed up as he was on so many different tablets and he has been discharged now. I don't know what to do.

Supervisor: Oh I wouldn't worry too much, the patient will probably have forgotten about what you told him by now, I am sure his GP will sort it all out.

In this example the supervisor does not know what to do and is unsure how to make a challenge, or indeed whether a challenge is needed, so therefore does nothing.

Supervisee: I feel I cannot take much more, it was such a tragedy, a loss of a life just like that. [There is a swell of tears and the supervisee is about to cry]
Supervisor: Do you want a hug? I find that often helps to help get over things like this?

Here, again, the supervisor does not know what to do and does not have the skill to enable and work through the catharsis with the supervisee.

Degenerative interventions are complex to understand and there are many forms and ways they can be delivered. The above is only a brief outline for raising awareness and bringing attention to the overall scope of this framework for personal development.

Conclusion

Having focused on a range of interventions for the clinical supervisor to use in all possible interactions with the supervisee, the next chapter will consider and explore a problem-solving framework. This will help give the supervisor structure and offer various skills and techniques when the task is to explore a problem, reach a new understanding and find solutions or goals.

Key learning points

- A competent and skilled supervisor should be able to identify a wide range of possible interventions that are effective and therapeutic when supervising.
- Being aware of different interventions for different needs helps the supervisor to become conscious of strengths and weaknesses in each of the six categories.
- Analysing how different interventions can elicit different responses and outcomes, the supervisor can act with a greater sense of purpose to benefit the supervisee and ultimately improve the care they provide.
- By developing skills within the six categories the supervisor will become a more effective therapist and will enable the supervisee to develop as a practitioner.
- A self-aware supervisor will recognize and therefore be able to steer away from the more degenerative forms of interventions.

7

A Problem-solving Framework
The skilled helper model

Chapter outcomes

By reading this chapter, doing the reflective activities, and integrating the material into your supervision practice, you should be able to

- Value and recognize the importance of a problem-solving framework.
- Understand the importance and value in facilitating problem solving.
- Recognize the importance of and possess some skills in problem solving.
- Recognize some key issues and skills in working towards solutions.
- Know about and possess some skills in focusing on the current scenario.
- Know about and possess some skills in focusing on the preferred scenario
- Know about and possess some skills in focusing on action strategies.
- Acknowledge and recognize the value of evaluation in a problem-solving framework.

Introduction

The framework presented here for problem solving is adapted from Egan (2002), who is probably among the best-known writers on helping skills. The 'skilled helper model', as it is usually referred to, is the most widely known counselling model in the world and extensively used in counselling training (Conner 1994). The terms used to describe the stages are taken from Egan

(2002), but I have adapted and tailored the content for the clinical supervisor to use when there is a need for exploration, reflection and taking action on issues which the supervisee brings to supervision. I feel that the model lends itself to supervision as it is reflective and follows a structure and process which can lead to new understanding and action.

Page and Wosket (1994) point out that supervision should always be exploratory if it is to be effective, and can be action orientated. The model is not based on any particular theory of personality development or of the ways in which difficulties develop. It is practical, can be simple but yet dynamic. It can also be viewed as an educative process as Egan (2002) maintains that helping should be a progression of learning that empowers the receiver to be their own source of problem solving. Nurses who are familiar with the nursing process may find some similarities with the stages and the shared responsibility of working together with the person who is receiving help. The process of evaluation, however, runs through and is fluid in all the stages, rather than its occurring at a specific juncture. Also similar to the nursing process, the underlying philosophy of approach is person centred.

Egan (2002) has defined the model as a framework as it provides a geographical map and outlines the tasks of helping and how they interrelate with each other. A model can be defined as a structure to help you get from A to B. A framework can be similarly defined but also considers and takes into account what you may need before you start, how to equip yourself with reserves and resources if things go wrong and how to evaluate at the conclusion. I will use the terms 'model' and 'framework' interchangeably as they both seem appropriate to use here. Egan (2002) makes it clear that this approach to problem solving is not all you ever wanted to know about helping. Keep an open mind and investigate other problem-solving models as well. With experience you will be able to make use of a variety of approaches and ideas and possibly integrate them into your own model. As this model is eclectic it lends itself well to the supervisor as a starting point for problem solving but also can be used and utilized in a flexible way. There are three stages to the model and three stages within the stages. The individual stages can be applied to many contexts that the supervisee brings to supervision and may be used independently and flexibly. Another advantage is that you may already have some of the skills necessary as they are transferable from everyday problem solving. Over time, the original terms used to describe the stages by Egan have been adapted and thus translated into more accessible terminology to suit the nature of the helping context. Wosket (2006) provides a comprehensive and balanced exposition of Egan's skilled helper model for those who wish to explore further.

The model is not theory based; instead, various methods and approaches to helping can be used in the framework. Egan (2002) does maintain and support the ideas of Carl Rogers that the core conditions of helping relationships (Chapter 3) are essential. However, unlike Rogers (1957), he veers away from their being sufficient, arguing that additional strategies and techniques are needed for helping to be effective.

The focus of the model is on solutions rather than problems. The emphasis is on discovering skills, strengths and resources to reach a preferred future outcome or goal, and whereby you are enabling the supervisee to manage their problems, develop their underused opportunities and to become more equipped to help themself (Egan 2002).

This skilled helper approach encourages the supervisee to become an active participant in the problem-solving process. Success usually comes when we, as human beings, are dynamic in initiating positive thinking and behaviour in order then to develop problem-solving strategies.

Reasons for a problem-solving model

The reason for this model in supervision is to provide a practical framework of helping, together with the skills and methods which make the model work. It can enable the supervisor to do the following:

- Have a map of knowing where to start when problem solving and directions of where to go next.
- Share the responsibility of problem solving.
- Explain the process as they move through the stages, so the supervisee knows and understands what is being done.
- Not always have the answers to problems, as all problems may not have answers or conclusions; yet with this model there is always something you can do, which is to listen and attend empathically.
- Work with the supervisee to acknowledge that success is not only about dealing with the problem but also staying in the solution.

For you as supervisor taking first steps, it is a matter of utilizing and developing your skills into a framework to give structure and direction. It will also offer insight in being able to more fully understand a problem-solving process, to recognize the value of the stages and to become more familiar with your supervisee. Fowler (2007) makes a case for solution-focused techniques to be used in clinical supervision which are adaptable to use in this framework. He states that the supervisor adopts a stance of a curious enquirer as you work through the process together. By communicating and demonstrating your interest in how the supervisee manages a particular situation, you have enabled the supervisee to acknowledge and identify their own abilities and skills in reaching a solution.

We will now consider the model (Figure 7.1) and then examine the individual stages and the application to helping the supervisee to solve problems in clinical supervision.

Not every supervisee will need to address all the individual stages. You may

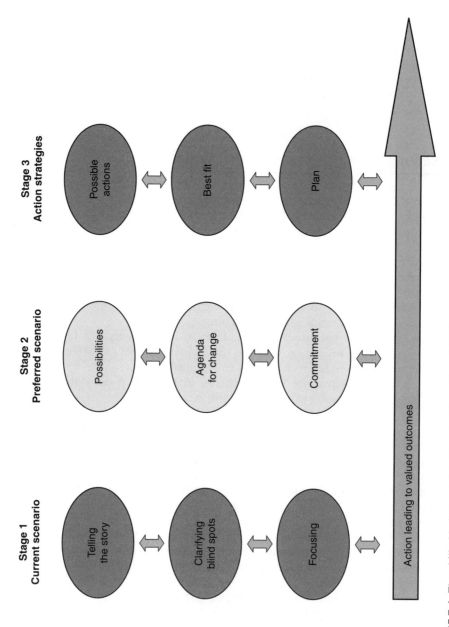

FIGURE 7.1 The skilled helper model. (Adapted from Egan 2002)

use each stage for its own merits or move back and forth as appropriate with your supervisee. It is, however, imperative that you are able to indentify your intention in what you are doing and why, and also that you are working with the supervisee, sharing those intentions to best fit their requirements for problem solving and personal development. To help you become familiar with the stages and the progression of the model I suggest you try the following reflective activity while reading through this chapter. You may want to work on your scenario using some of, if not all of, the different parts of the stages. This will help you to integrate the framework into practice and become more familiar with it when using it with your supervisee.

Reflective activity

Note down a current issue or problem you have at work, one that involves you and that you have some control and responsibility to change or make better. For example, a current problem situation that involves your clinical practice; a problem situation that involves you and others in your role as a healthcare worker; an aspect of yourself, perhaps it is one that you know holds you back, that you wish to develop in order to become more accomplished as a healthcare worker.

To have a brief overview of the framework and process, consider the three overall stages (Figure 7.1). With your problem situation in mind, make some brief notes, starting with stage 1, using the question below.

Stage 1: The current scenario. Ask yourself: 'What is going on?', or 'What is not working as well as it could?'

As you read through the three stages in this chapter, apply the suggested materials to your own problem scenario and make notes as you progress through stages 2 and 3.

Stage 2: The preferred scenario. Ask yourself: 'What do I want and need?' or 'What solutions or goals do I want to achieve?'

Stage 3: Action strategies. Ask yourself: 'What strategies can I make and plan for to achieve my goals?'

This framework can be used on your own problems and for self-supervision. It can help you to indentify your goals and to pursue them.

However, for it to be used to its most beneficial and for the most advantage it requires the objectiveness and skill of a helper. Such a helper, as you are beginning to learn, will be able to enable that process, through support, challenge, facilitating exploration, and clarification by helping you move forward with your shared and verbal commitment to action.

Stage 1. The current scenario or problem situation

Overview of stage 1

A question being asked in this stage is 'what is going on?' The answer to that question will constitute the current problem situation. The focus here is on exploring the presenting issues or concerns. There may be several major components to the issue, making matters rather complex and seemingly unmanageable. Your task is to help screen out the less significant issues and focus on the main thoughts, feeling and behaviours, prioritize and then concentrate on the particular issue that the supervisee wants to work on first. Undeveloped or missed opportunities may be brought to the attention of the supervisee. These terms used by Egan (2002) refer to the personal resources and opportunities that the person is not developing. By defining and exploring the unreached potential in the supervisee you can engender more creativity and enable them to function more fully, both professionally and personally. Stage 1 is shown in Figure 7.2 along with its specific stages.

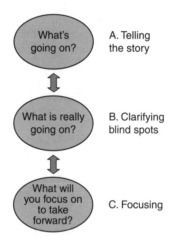

FIGURE 7.2 Stage 1: the current scenario

Stage 1A. Telling the story: what's going on

The task of stage 1A is to help your supervisee begin to talk about the problem or issue they wish to solve. Your supervisees will differ in their ability and willingness to talk about the issue and, in particular, what is going on beneath the surface, if indeed they are aware of what that is. A mix of active listening, empathy and probing are basic tools and requirements for both clarity and disclosing of issues.

Some appropriate questions to ask

- Where would you like to start?
- How do you see the current scenario?
- What exactly is your role and responsibility within the situation?
- What are your thoughts and feelings about it?
- What are your concerns?
- Which particular aspect has the most importance for you?
- What has the most importance for your clients? For your colleagues?
- What are you able to take responsibility for so that you can begin to look for change?

The above open questions would begin to help your supervisee to focus on the issue that they wish to resolve. The next interventions are more probing and clarifying, to help your supervisee to explore a little deeper. For example:

- 'So you seem to being saying . . . Is that right?'
- 'What is holding you back from where you want to be and doing what you want to do?'
- 'Can I just clarify that point, what do you actually mean when you say . . .?'
- 'What skills and resources do you have, but perhaps underuse?'
- 'What could you accomplish if you put your mind to it?'
- 'What opportunities are there for you?'
- 'So, to help bring this into focus, let us summarize the main issues/points.'

By having built a helping and empathic relationship you are able to provide a safe place for the supervisee to tell their story or problem. The aim is to help explore and unfold the presenting problem so the supervisee can hear and understand themselves and gain a clearer picture. It is important here to focus on the story and not the history. If we don't know what to do and where to go with the story, it is tempting to look for more detail. Unlike other clinical or professional roles you may have, your role here is not to take a full history. As time is limited we need to focus and sift out the relevant facts and have a question in our own minds of is this story moving forward?' (Egan 2002). Your aim is to help the supervisee to talk about those aspects which are infringing on the presenting problem. Make the full use of your time by focusing on the issues that are present now and are affecting performance.

While helping supervisees to talk through their problem there will be openings to help them reflect on unused or missed opportunities. Egan (2002) refers to these as blind spots. By helping your supervisee to explore and clarify their problem situation and unexploited opportunities, past and present, the aim is to enable better understanding. This is in order to eventually reach a conclusion or goal and to have a different perspective on the situation.

Solutions are not always about dealing with the problem, as problems do not always have answers. By listening to the issue the supervisee is bringing, you begin to gain understanding and they to gain a clearer picture of the situation.

Stage 1B. Clarifying blind spots: what is really going on

The task of stage 1B is to uncover or challenge areas that may be hindering the awareness of your supervisee. Egan (2002) uses the term 'blind spots' to refer to the areas to challenge. This is related to the blind area of the Johari Window (Chapter 3). The purpose of challenge and constructive feedback here is to raise awareness in the supervisee on aspects of themselves that they are relatively unaware of. These aspects are holding them back from achieving more of their potential and reaching the goals they want to achieve. A blind spot can be a weak spot that is holding them back or strengths that they are reluctant or refusing to acknowledge. This can be through lack of knowledge, insight, misunderstanding or refusal to see another's point of view. A general principle here when challenging is to help the supervisee to develop new perspectives, take control and ownership of the issue and move forward.

Some common areas to challenge

Not owning the problem: blaming and avoiding 'I' language
Generally, when we avoid owning the problem there is a tendency to rationalize, meaning to make excuses or to project and blame others. By using phrases such 'everyone feels that way' or 'anyone would', we avoid owning the problem and saying 'I'. This is a way of distancing ourselves from the situation and our feelings. A suggested response and challenge to the supervisee could be: 'You are saying anyone would, I am wondering if you could rephrase that by saying how you would feel?'

Vagueness
Another method of distancing or avoiding what is really going on is stating problems in a vague way or being ambiguous. Such comments need clarification. Here are three examples:

- 'It was just a crazy situation.'
  Supervisor response: 'You say crazy, what do you actually mean by crazy?'
- 'I'm always rubbish at doing that.'
  Supervisor response: 'Always?' If offered in a soft but challenging tone this has the effect of being reflective rather than asking a direct question.
- 'Anyone would get angry about the mess things are in.'
  Supervisor response: 'What you really mean is you can get angry about this current situation. What in particular makes you feel that way?'

Blaming people, places or things
We may hear comments from the supervisee that put the blame elsewhere. For example:

- 'She made me feel so angry that's why I shouted.'
  Suggested supervisor response: 'You are feeling angry and lost your temper.'
- 'They should stop giving me all that stress to deal with.'
  Supervisor response: 'You're recognizing some level of stress for yourself at the moment, which is important, how about us looking at some ways to address that?'
- 'With my workload it's impossible to eat sensibly or take any kind of break during the day.'
  Supervisor response: 'Okay, take a moment to think about what you just said, because I know you do consider things carefully, what could be some consequences for you?'

While staying supportive you are challenging the supervisee to view themself in relation to the problem and own the feeling. You are helping to uncover a blind spot that, if brought to their notice, would enable them to take ownership of the issue. Using skills such as paraphrasing, clarifying and summarizing, the above statements can be reflected back to the supervisee in the form of a challenge.

Having little or no choice
When your supervisee is using words such as 'should', 'can't', or 'must' then they may be indicating that there is no real choice or that there is some compulsion or pressure to sort something out. That may well be the case, but it may help to raise awareness and challenge that belief. Other powerful words such as 'always' and 'never' are sometimes used to indicate that the situation is absolute or definite and beyond any change of thinking. Here are three examples:

- 'What's the point? I can't do it.'
  Supervisor response: 'I am wondering when you say can't whether you mean won't. Perhaps it's worth exploring what is stopping you?'
- 'I have never been able to be assertive; it has always been that way.'
  Supervisor response: 'Never is rather a strong word you are using. Knowing you as I do, you do not shy away from learning new tasks. I am wondering if part of you is avoiding something.'
  I learnt from a previous supervisor to use the phrase 'part of you' at times when making a challenge or giving feedback on aspects of change. 'Part of you' makes the issue sound less gigantic and therefore more manageable; resolution seems more achievable if the problem belongs to only part of you.
- 'I should be able to adapt but I don't take to change very well.'

Supervisor response: 'If you were to say I could choose to adapt, instead of I should, how would that sound to you?'

Helping the supervisee to change words from 'should' to 'could' and to choose, puts the issue in a different frame. You are enabling thoughts to become clearer, feelings are owned and you are inviting choice.

Helping your supervisee to reflect specifically on what they are saying can uncover certain blind areas, as the above examples demonstrate. Only when the problem or issue is owned can you help the supervisee to move forward to a solution which will be realistic and potentially solvable.

Some questions that can offer a challenge

- 'What issues are there for you that you are avoiding?'
- 'You may be overlooking something; if you were, what would that be?'
- 'I'm wondering what part of you blocks that.'
- 'In what specific way can you verify that assumption?'
- 'If you had been observing yourself, what would you have noticed?'
- 'What feedback have you been given in the past and, in being honest with yourself, was rather difficult to take on board?'
- 'The way I see you in that situation is rather different, perhaps you under-value yourself when you . . . Would that be a fair comment?

Challenge is used in the context here as an invitation for the supervisee to find a new perspective on their situation.

Highlighting discrepancies in what the supervisee is saying can speed up the helping process and overcome a block or barrier. Challenges are best presented in a tentative manner but not in such a way that they lack assertiveness.

Summarizing as a challenging skill

You can use summarizing as a challenging skill when you are pulling together themes of the blocks the supervisee puts on their performance or progress. You have observed these over time from your discussions and they are becoming a familiar pattern. By summarizing you could point out, for example, that the supervisee does not fully use the resources or opportunities that come their way, or that there have been several situations in clinical practice where perhaps they have acted on impulse rather than thinking the problem through. In isolation those situations may be minor, but as a pattern could result in significant learning for your supervisee. Remember when summarizing and the intention is to challenge, there needs to be a balance of the supervisee's strengths to ensure the focus is not all on the negatives.

Stage 1C. Focusing: what to take forward

The task of stage 1C is to help your supervisee to focus and to prioritize where to start. They may be grappling with many issues at the same time and feel stuck. The issues may feel too big or overwhelming or they are intertwined and convoluted. This stage helps to manage this perplexity and aims to move the supervisee from 'stuckness' to hope. You help your supervisee identify major concerns, especially if there is a range of issues, to come to decisions and choose which problems or opportunities to work on first and which will make a difference. This may involve screening out the less significant parts of the story so that the important issues can be looked at. You help your supervisee to prioritize, for example, which issue, if managed successfully, will help contribute to the success of the other issues. You may also need to break down the whole problem into smaller parts so that it becomes more manageable.

Questions to help focus

- 'What, of all that we have talked about so far, is most important to you?'
- 'What do you think would be best to work on now?'
- 'Which or what would make the most difference?'
- 'Which problem, if worked on, will help the other problems?'
- 'What is the most manageable problem for you?'

Some principles when focusing

- Handle any crisis first.
- Focus on what is most important to the supervisee.
- Begin with the problem that is causing the most concern or stress.
- Begin with a manageable sub-problem.
- Begin with the problem that shows the most promise of success.
- Begin with the problem that will lead to a general improvement.
- Begin with the less difficult and then move on to the more difficult problems.
- Focus on the problem where the benefits will be high and the costs low.

The objectives of stage 1 have been met when a rapport has been established and the supervisee has explored a problem they wish to solve or move forward with. Clarifying and challenge can enable the supervisee to take full responsibility for the task they are to set themself. Blind areas may have been uncovered that are central to the problem; the supervisee has reflected on unconscious factors that are involved so a greater understanding and awareness is gained. Having a clearer view, the supervisee can begin to identify and choose where to start and the opportunities to work on. For some supervisees, talking through their story and simply being heard may be enough in itself and you both may choose to leave it there; for others this may just be the beginning and you move on to the next stage.

Reflective activity

In the previous reflective activity you were asked to identify a current work-related issue or problem that you wished to solve. Having read through stage 1, work through the following questions related to the specific stages.

1A Have you gained any clarity regarding the current situation?
1B Although it is a contradiction to be aware of your own blind spots, are you aware of any of the blocks that hold you back from making further progress or that hinder your development? Which do you need to work on to enable you to move forward with this current issue?
1C Have you been able to focus on and prioritize a particular (if there were several) issue to start with?

Stage 2. The preferred scenario

Overview of stage 2

A question being asked in stage 2 is 'what do you really want?' A first step is to explore the possibilities of change and to consider a range of options. From these a viable agenda is focused on, along with new understandings of and perspectives on the situation. This helps the supervisee to make choices, set achievable goals and look forward to the difference the changes can make. There is opportunity in this stage to help your supervisee to use their imagination and creativity to map out a better situation or future of what they want and need. Stage 2 is shown in Figure 7.3 along with its specific stages.

Stage 2A. Being creative: possibilities

Having gained an understanding of either the problem situation or the opportunities for development, the task of this next stage is to assist your supervisee to envisage how the situation could be if it were better, and to begin to look for solutions. A range of possibilities is first considered to develop awareness and potential for finding those solutions. I offer below some suggestions of how questions can be asked that focus on possibilities for change.

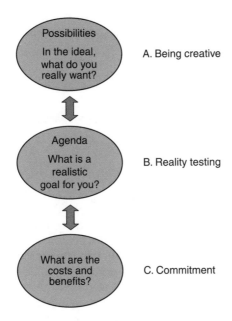

FIGURE 7.3 Stage 2: the preferred scenario

Some appropriate questions for exploring possibilities for change

- What do you ideally want or would like instead?
- What would be happening?
- What would you be doing, thinking, feeling?
- What would it [the preferred situation] look like?
- Imagine if it were different; how would it be?
- Well, let's look first at what you do not want, and then we may be able to focus on what you do want.
- What would you have that you don't have now?
- What would be a noticeable change in you?
- What would others notice that was different?

Word-storming can also be used to assist the supervisee to think creatively and divergently. Divergent thinking is useful here because often in problem situations, and in particular when dealing with the supervisee's feelings, thinking and behaviour, there will be no right or wrong answer. Edward de Bono (1992) uses the term 'lateral thinking'. He viewed creativity in human thinking as a most human resource, to avoid forever repeating the same patterns and to be able to progress. We aim here to develop our supervisee in their thinking and to be open to the view that there is more than one way to manage a problem or develop an opportunity.

Some key points when word-storming to facilitate imaginative thinking

- Quantity of ideas rather than quality of ideas.
- Suspend judgement, both of you.
- Anything goes, so go wild and have fun.
- Avoid analysis.
- Keep prompting, 'what else?' and 'that's good; any more ideas?'
- Use one idea to create and stimulate another.
- Allow time, do not hurry.

Stage 2B. Reality testing: agenda for change

Following on from generating the creative and visionary ideas in considering the possibilities, the task of stage 2B includes helping the supervisee to choose which of those ideas are specific, measurable, appropriate and realistic. The aim here is to help choose one or more of those possibilities that can be turned into goals for constructive change. This agenda for change needs to be workable, for it is later to be converted into action. While goals are being identified we need to check that they are within the values, capabilities and resources of the supervisee.

SMART goals

A well used and simple approach to setting goals is known by the acronym SMART. A SMART goal is a goal that is:

Specific
Measurable
Achievable (or Appropriate or Agreed upon)
Realistic (or Rewardable)
Time framed

When working with your supervisee on setting goals, there may be no need to work through all the criteria of SMART. This will depend on their resourcefulness, experience and skills. The approach can be used in a variety of supervision contexts where a focus is on achievement and setting of goals. Have a look at the following SMART suggestions.

Specific

A specific goal has a much greater chance of being accomplished than a general goal. The less vague you are when devising goals the more chance of success. Try to get your supervisee to be specific so they begin to know exactly what they want and need.

To set a specific goal, ask some of the following questions:

- What do you want to accomplish?
- Where is it going to happen?
- When is it going to happen?
- What are the specific reasons for wanting to accomplish this goal?
- Who is going to be involved?
- What resources will you need?
- Will it be clear to the relevant others?

Measurable
Establish a criterion that is real and tangible against which progress towards each goal can be measured. Ask questions such as:

- How will you know when you have achieved it?
- How will you know when it has been accomplished?

Achievable (or Appropriate or Agreed upon)
To plan goals wisely, help the supervisee explore and develop their attitudes, abilities, values and skills that they may need. Of importance here is consideration of values and beliefs. Aims, goals and future action need to be within the value system of the supervisee, both personally and, more importantly, professionally within the organization for which they are working. Ask questions such as:

- What do you need that will help?
- What are you able to manage?
- What are you likely to achieve?
- Who else is it going to affect?
- Is this goal within your, and others', value system?

Reaching agreement that the goal is appropriate and achievable can help build self-esteem, which enables the move into action. Offer feedback to your supervisee that they are worthy of these goals and give encouragement so that they develop the traits needed to in order to achieve them. When your supervisee knows that they can be achieved you can begin to work out the next steps to attaining them.

Realistic (or Rewarding)
To be realistic, a goal must represent an objective towards which you are willing and able to work. The goal is probably realistic if you truly believe that it can be accomplished and that you have the resources. Ask questions such as:

- Have you accomplished anything similar in the past?
- What conditions need to exist to accomplish this goal?
- What are you going to need?
- What resources are you going to need?

A goal can be both challenging and realistic. Your supervisee can only really decide how challenging the goal should be, but remind them that every goal represents substantial progress. Often, a more challenging goal increases the motivation to achieve it, whereas an easily achieved goal exerts only a low motivational force. A goal, however, needs to be both realistic and rewarding and within the reach of the supervisee's skills, qualities, talents and circumstances.

Time framed
A goal should be grounded within a realistic time frame, for if no time frame is set there may be no sense of urgency or motivation to achieve the goal. Rather than allowing your supervisee to set goals 'someday soon' or 'when I get around to it', ask such questions as the following as they help to set the mind into motion and are more specific:

- When do you want to achieve this by?
- Does that give you enough time?
- How do you know?

Stage 2C. Commitment: costs and benefits

The task of stage 2C is to test the realism of the goal, which is a further dimension of the goal-setting process. It also checks out the commitment to the goal by reviewing the costs and benefits to the supervisee (and others) of achieving it. The previous stage of clearly identifying goals will generally fail if the goals are not going to be actively pursued by the supervisee.

Some suggested questions to ask on commitment

- Which of the identified goals have the greatest priority or are the most urgent?
- What will be the benefits and advantages when you achieve this?
- How will you be different?
- What will be the costs? For example, can you see any disadvantages or downsides in doing this?
- How might it affect others?
- How do you really feel about the choice and decision you are going to take?
- Are you making this choice freely?
- What are the incentives and rewards?
- How committed are you to carrying this out?
- How hard will you work at it?
- How will you stay committed?

In summary, stage 2 provides the opportunities to explore how the goal or change is to take shape for the better. By being creative in exploring options and possibilities and then focusing on what is achievable, the commitment is likely to be more realistic. Remember, this stage is about what the supervisee wants or needs to accomplish, but not necessarily, yet, how they will accomplish it.

Reflective activity

Following on from the previous activity, work through these questions regarding stage 2.

2A What would my preferred scenario be like and how would it look if it was better?

2B What realistically will be possible and achievable? You may want to use the SMART goals to help you.

2C Have you considered the consequences and do the benefits outweigh any costs? How committed are you in going ahead with a plan?

Stage 3. Action strategies

Overview of stage 3

This final stage is about action. A question being asked is 'what strategies can you make and plan for to achieve your goals?' Working through stage 3 will help produce strategies for implementing a plan of action to reach achievable and realistic goals. Stage 3 is shown in Figure 7.4 overleaf along with its specific stages.

Stage 3A. Possible actions: strategies and plans

Now that a choice of goal or accomplishment has been made, the task of stage 3A is to identify the actions you could take to achieve it.

Energy and hope can be felt by your supervisee as the focus becomes the goals and accomplishments rather than the problem. Egan (2002: 248) states this succinctly as: '*Goals, not problems, should drive action.*'

Word-storming can again be used to generate ideas and then plans to reach the outcomes or goals. Remember, there is usually more than one way to achieve a goal.

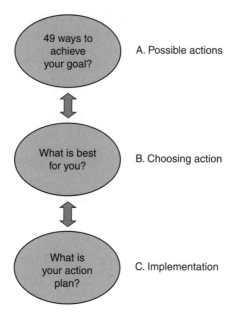

FIGURE 7.4 Stage 3: action strategies

Some suggested questions to identify possible actions

- What are all the different ways you can go about this?
- How else might you go about this task?
- What do you know has worked for others?
- What are all the ways you can get started?
- What skills and resources do you need before you begin?
- Who or what else will help you?

Stage 3B. Choosing the best-fit action

The task of stage 3B is to choose which of the action strategies is the most realistic and suitable as we consider the best way forward in attempting to achieve the desired outcome for the presenting problem.

Some suggested questions for deciding best-fit actions

- Which of the ideas and strategies appeal to you the most?
- Which will help you to achieve what you need?
- Which would be best for this situation?

- Which are within your resources and control?
- Which are within your value system?
- What will be the benefits?
- What will be the costs?
- What will help and hinder you in achieving your goal?

When a workable plan has been formulated the next and final stage will be for your supervisee to act. One method of helping them to prepare to act is to identify the factors that will help or hinder the implementation of the goal. A technique to use for this process is called force field analysis.

Force field analysis

Force field analysis is perhaps an awkward name given to a very useful and simple technique. Devised by the psychologist Kurt Lewin (1890–1947), it can be used as a method of decision making when planning and implementing change. Its name refers to the forces or factors that can influence that implementation. There are forces that may help and there are forces that may hinder. When applied to decision making it can more simply be described as weighing up the pros and cons. The method is suitable here when planning goals in supervision and when focusing on action plans to introduce change. The general question being asked to the supervisee is, 'what will increase the chances or opportunities of this plan starting, working and fulfilling the intended outcomes, and what may decrease the chances?' For example, what are the driving or facilitating forces for change and what are the blocking or restraining forces that are working against it?

The force field diagram (Figure 7.5 overleaf) is built on the idea that forces are both driving and restraining change. These forces, represented by the arrows in Figure 7.5, can and will include people, places and things as well as your own resources, rules, costs, habits, attitudes and so on. When working with this formula the idea is to identify and acknowledge the principal forces that are going to help you and the principal forces that will hinder you (Egan 1985). The arrows that push upwards represent the driving forces; these are to be positive and you want them to grow. The arrows pointing down represent the restraining forces; these are negative and you want them to diminish. The force field analysis diagram may help you to picture the fight between the forces around a given issue.

There are the several steps which you can talk your supervisee through when working with force field analysis:

1 Describe the desired goal or situation.
2 List all the forces that would help and facilitate change to the desired situation. Think in terms of self, people, places and things.

Restraining forces that impede progress and cause failure

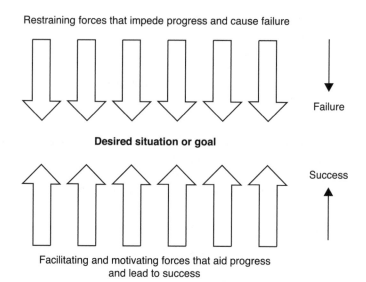

Desired situation or goal

Success

Facilitating and motivating forces that aid progress
and lead to success

FIGURE 7.5 Force field analysis

3 List all the forces hindering or restraining changes towards the desired situation. Think in terms of self, people, places and things.
4 Discuss and question all the forces. Ask: are they valid? Can they be changed? Which are strong and which are weak?
5 Explore how to reduce the strength and number of the restraining forces.
6 Explore how to increase the strength and number of helping forces.
7 Remember that increasing the helping forces and decreasing the hindering forces may have a knock-on effect with others or even create new ones.
8 Make a note of actions to be taken for the desired changes to the any of the forces.

Force field analysis is a useful technique for looking at all the forces for and against a plan. By weighing up the importance of these factors you can decide whether the plan is workable or whether any changes are needed to improve it. Having completed this very necessary process, you can begin the implementation of the plan.

Stage 3C. Implementation: the action plan

The task in this final stage is to as accurately as possible help the supervisee plan the implementation of an action plan. The strategy for action is broken down into bite-size chunks or manageable components and you are helping to turn good intentions and commitments into a specific plan.

Some suggested questions for implementing the plan

- What is your first step?
- Is there anything you need to do before taking the first step?
- How will you gather together the resources you need?
- What will be the next step?
- Whom do you need to inform?
- Where is this to happen?
- When is it to take place?
- In what order are these activities to take place?
- How flexible do you want to be with your plan?

In summary, stage 3 explores the possible action plans and solutions. The best-fit strategies and ideas that are to be most beneficial are considered, in fine detail if need be, for the supervisee then to choose and construct a plan of action.

Reflective activity

Following on from the previous activity, work through these questions regarding stage 3.

3A What strategies have you considered and explored in helping to make your plan workable?

3B What plan are you going to go ahead with?

3C How exactly, step by step, are you going to implement the plan?

Some final thoughts

Having read and worked through the model it may help to note that the A, B and C stages within each stage tend to have a similar intention:

- The A stages are exploratory.
- The B stages are for checking out.
- The C stages are for focusing and committing.

When this model is used in supervision, it can, and needs to, be flexible. Unlike in counselling, you are not solving personal problems and do not have as much time. In supervision you are dealing primarily with healthcare-related issues of a professional nature. Therefore you are able to use each stage, and each stage within a stage, independently and to apply each as appropriate to the supervisee's needs and situation. If, however, you find yourself stuck or going round in circles, reflect on the stage you are in and why: you will probably find that you have missed out important steps along the way or have moved too far ahead too soon. A tendency in helpers who are not familiar with facilitating the process of helping others to achieve their own change, is to jump from the problem to action. Too often exploration and clarification of problem situations is followed immediately by planning action, without a clear, considered and realistic idea of the desired goal or outcome. To put this in terms of the framework, it is to jump from stage 1 to stage 3. As a result, the action plan usually fails at some point as there is a shortfall in the real commitment and resources needed. Options to help stimulate, encourage and motivate have possibly not been explored. These would not then have been clarified, assessed and truly focused on.

Remember to evaluate and summarize as you move through or use each stage. Explain what you are doing and why to your supervisee. By sharing the methods in this overall plan, the task has been shared. There is no mystical way you have been working; your supervisee is more able to perform the action plan, as it is theirs, not something that has been suggested from your expertise, or indeed conjured up. By sharing the techniques and procedures you are enabling the supervisee to empower themself even more and they can then apply some of the skills to their own helping activities when and where appropriate.

Egan (2002) highlights the need for the helper to keep an evaluative eye on the entire process and to have a sense and feel for the severity of the problem and the ability the person has in handling it. Those sentiments do transfer to the supervision process. You are there for the benefit of the supervisee and do have a role in keeping an eye on their delivery of healthcare. Although this is not a managerial responsibility as such, as you are not acting as their line manager, you do have a responsibility for their well-being and well-doing as a healthcare worker. So always, within this framework, there needs to be an evaluative eye on the process and projected outcomes.

Conclusion

When an action plan or change of practice has been implemented it is valuable for the supervisee to reflect in order to learn from the experience and make any further changes. The next chapter will focus on reflective practice and consider a model to use for this purpose.

Key learning points

- A skilled supervisor is able to structure a problem-solving process by having a plan to follow that is tailored to the needs of the individual.
- A supervisor strengthens the facilitating process with empathic listening and responding and shares with the supervisee an evaluative eye on decisions and projected outcomes.
- Over time and with practice a supervisor will be able to move more flexibly through the stages of problem solving and integrate specific stages to accommodate the supervisee's specific wants and needs.
- However, a skilled supervisor always knows the direction and intention of the skills and techniques they are using.
- Good quality problem solving is about helping the supervisee to develop new understanding of the problems and working towards solutions and not jumping in straight away with finding the solution or making a decision for them.
- A skilled supervisor understands and is developing the skills of exploring, challenging and focusing while working in stage 1 of the problem-solving framework with the supervisee.
- A skilled supervisor, when moving into stage 2, helps the supervisee to develop creative skills and looks at a range of possibilities and outcomes.
- A supervisor has the skills of facilitating the supervisee to consider a first range of strategies to achieve the goal before a decision is reached, by understanding this, the supervisor can help shape the action plan and implementation.

8

Reflective Practice and the Supervisor

Chapter outcomes

By reading this chapter, doing the reflective activities, and integrating the material into your supervision practice, you should be able to:

- Define and have some understanding of the concept of reflective practice.
- Recognize the similarities between reflective practice and clinical supervision.
- Acknowledge the value of reflective practice for clinical supervision.
- Become familiar with a reflective practice cycle.
- Know about and possess some cue questions to use in the stages of a reflective cycle.

Introduction

There is an abundance of literature on reflective practice for healthcare professionals and several models and frameworks to use for purposeful and structured reflection. This area is rapidly growing and it is not within the scope of this book to cover reflective practice in any more depth than I do here. What I do intend to present is some understanding of the importance and significance of reflective practice for use in clinical supervision and a model to use. Gibbs's (1988) reflective cycle is detailed as one of several that are available and transferable to a supervision context. I will offer a practical introduction to the model, considering its benefits and application to clinical supervision.

Defining reflective practice

There are many definitions of reflective practice. The word 'reflection' is widely used in teaching, education, coaching and the healthcare professions. The term has many connotations; I have chosen a few that indicate its implications and usefulness for supervision. They are:

- To ponder
- To consider
- To contemplate
- To muse
- To mull over
- To suggest
- To indicate
- To evaluate

First, it is important to differentiate between reflection and reflective practice. Kottkamp (1990) defines reflective practice as *'a mode that links thought and action with reflection, it involves clinically analysing one's actions with the goal of improving one's professional practice'*. However, reflection as defined by Boud et al. (1985) is *'an activity in which people recapture their experience, think about it, mull over it and evaluate it'*.

We can see here that reflection is only a part of reflective practice; another view is that reflective practice is an extension of reflection. We may be able to develop the skills to reflect for improved understanding but that does not necessarily mean it will improve our practice. Reflective practice is the application of those skills with the aim and focus to improve practice. The point I am making is that clinical supervision is a vehicle for both; it is a place to reflect and a means by which the learning and understanding can be applied to practice. I will refer to both aspects of reflection interchangeably, as ultimately the aim is to improve practice.

You may wish to think of reflection for supervision as a mirror, to look at yourself and what you have been doing. Schön (1983) proposes that the process depends on two types of reflection:

- Reflection in action
- Reflection on action

Reflection in action means noticing and examining your own and others' behaviour while in the situation and at the time it happens. Reflection on action takes place after the event and is perhaps the more common form. It involves looking back, reviewing and then evaluating the positives and negatives with a view to improving practice and being more effective in the future.

Experience in reflecting *on* action will facilitate the more advanced skills and expertise of reflecting *in* action. A good example of where reflection on action would take place is clinical supervision, and you are in position here to develop the skills and qualities in your supervisee so that they can begin to develop reflection in action.

Reflective practice in clinical supervision

There are many similarities between reflective practice and supervision. More than a decade ago Fisher (1996) pointed out the links between the two and the majority of literature on clinical supervision will acknowledge or concentrate on the relationship between reflective practice and supervision. From the literature there are several themes that emerge regarding the similarities; these are listed in the box below.

Similarities between reflective practice and clinical supervision

- Improving practice
- Professional development
- Continuing education
- Readiness to change
- Learning from experience
- Understanding experiences
- Looking backwards and forwards
- Thoughtful deliberation
- Being open honest with yourself
- Being self-aware
- Self-enquiry
- Questioning routine or habitual practice
- Challenging conventional thinking and wisdom
- Creative thinking
- Evaluating
- Implementing learning
- Taking action

A fundamental similarity between the two concepts is the willingness to develop, learn, change and improve practice. The relationship between reflective practice and clinical supervision can be viewed in two ways. Clinical supervision can be seen as a contracted and agreed formal process in which supervisees can engage in reflection, and reflective practice can be seen as an essential part of supervision. A supervisee can make effective use of reflective practice as a learning tool within the context of supervision and this can be guided by frameworks and reflective cycles. Many of the skills and qualities already identified in this book as necessary for a supervisor can be used to facilitate the reflective supervisee. Gillings (2000) states that prerequisites are the commitment to the process and a shared understanding to make the experience of reflection effective. Boyd and Fales (1983) also strongly suggest the value of self-development when developing reflective practice.

It could be argued that good supervisors are by definition reflective practitioners and, hopefully, good ones. I suggest that this will be the case if the supervisor constantly strives to improve their own practice, through reflection and supervision and therefore becoming an honest and genuine role model to their supervisees. Jasper (2006) summarizes the benefits of having a reflective practitioner in the workforce; these can be seen in the box below.

Benefits arising from reflective practice

Practising reflectively results in benefits for:

- The individual, in terms of providing individualized care, identifying their learning needs, and learning from experience.
- The patient, in terms of higher quality and standards of care, and care designed to meet their own unique needs.
- The employer, in terms of standards of care achieved, in having a continually developing workforce which recognizes its own professional development needs.
- The profession, in terms of self-regulation of the practitioners, in developing nurses' knowledge base, in contributing to increasing the status of nursing and recognition of nurses' contribution to patient care.

Source: Jasper 2006

All the benefits listed in the box would be as equally relevant to the benefits of clinical supervision. Jasper (2006) makes out a strong case for the continuing development and recognition of reflective practitioners and it would seem to me that clinical supervision would be an ideal forum where reflection can take place. The skills and qualities of the supervisor can provide a legitimate, formal and structured learning opportunity for the supervisee to reflect on their practice. It would also be twofold, as both parties can develop skills of reflective practice in aiming for the benefits as described in the box. As a supervisor, you develop reflective practice in your own supervision and you facilitate reflective practice with your supervisees.

In order to develop and learn reflective practice in clinical supervision it will help to have a framework to begin with.

Reasons for a reflective framework

Although a framework of reflection is not essential, it can provide a useful starting point, by aiding self-development, commitment and understanding, therefore helping to put reflection into action. Platzer et al. (1997) identify that learning through reflection is greater if there is understanding of frameworks that provide a structural process.

There are many published frameworks for reflection, and Jasper (2006) identifies, analyses and compares some of the most popular. From these I have chosen the framework of Gibbs (1988) because it is generic and user friendly. It is widely known in the healthcare professions so you may already be familiar with the format. It also used widely in educational settings (Palmer et al. 1994). It is straightforward to use, adaptable and flexible.

When choosing a framework it is important that the supervisor and supervisee understand what they are trying to achieve and the purpose that the framework will have for supervision. Ask first what the supervisee understands by reflective practice, how they see the benefits, and their experience of using frameworks or other techniques. Work and agree together on a framework and how this may be employed, discussing the stages of reflection with reference to a particular framework. This last point is important, as otherwise it is possible that both parties will aim for different outcomes by implementing slightly different variations of a reflective framework.

A model of reflection

Gibbs's (1988) experiential learning cycle involves reflection as a key element and provides a framework to guide the reflection and to learn from the experience. I feel it is applicable and adaptable to the helping professions as it does recognize both thoughts and feelings, and it values evaluation, analysis and implementing plans of action: all essential components for the supervisee to focus on, as the emphasis of the framework, and clinical supervision, is on development, learning and improvement of practice. The objective of Gibbs's reflective cycle in supervision is for your supervisee to learn from the experiences that they bring to supervision from their practice. Although reflective practice often involves reviewing or contemplating a negative experience with a view to improving practice, it can also be used to celebrate positive experiences with a view to developing strengths in order to improve even further, as it encourages the evolution of new ideas. The model can be seen in Figure 8.1.

The cycle starts at the top of the diagram with a description of what happened, moving on to focusing on the supervisee's feelings and then evaluation

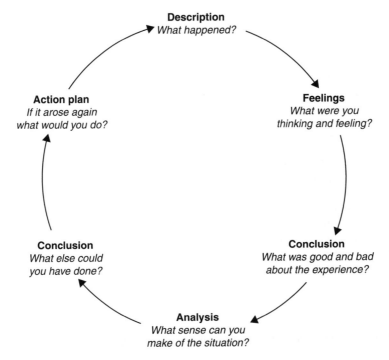

Description
What happened?

Action plan
*If it arose again
what would you do?*

Feelings
*What were you
thinking and feeling?*

Conclusion
*What else could
you have done?*

Conclusion
*What was good and bad
about the experience?*

Analysis
*What sense can you
make of the situation?*

FIGURE 8.1 A reflective cycle. (Gibbs 1988)

of what was good and bad. Analysis follows and then conclusions are drawn, leading on to making an action plan. The focus or perspective of the framework is on continuous learning and development and is particularly useful for contributing to a change in practice, as the cycle can be used after the action plan has been implemented to aid reflection again on that changed practice.

There are suggested cue questions to be asked at each stage, although guard against treating these as a set of instructions or a checklist. View them more as prompts and starting points. I will present here the stages in more detail along with some suggested cue questions. There are many similarities with Johns's (2004) model, which is another popular reflective framework, so therefore I have taken the opportunity to integrate some of those questions into the framework being presented here.

Description: What happened?

In this stage you are helping your supervisee to describe the event in detail and objectively. This is a situation they want to reflect on and learn more about, so it is important at first that they take a step back and view it as if they were an outside observer.

You are helping your supervisee not only to describe the event in detail but also to consider it and pick up on aspects of the situation that they did not consider at the time. Helping your supervisee to look at their responses and the responses of others can help when you focus on how they would approach a similar situation again. However, while at this stage of describing what happened you both need to stay objective and avoid making judgements; nor should you draw any conclusions as yet.

Useful cue questions are:

- What was the context of the event; why were you there?
- What happened?
- Who else was there?
- What were you doing?
- How did you respond?
- What were other people doing?
- What was your part in this?
- What parts did the other people play?
- What was the result?

Feelings/reactions: What were you thinking and feeling?

In this stage you are helping your supervisee to both focus on and explore their thoughts and feelings at the time of the situation they have been describing.

Useful cue questions are:

- How you were feeling when the event started?
- What you were thinking about at the time?
- How did it make you feel?
- What feelings did others evoke in you?
- How do you think the others felt? How did you know this?
- How did you feel about the outcome of the event?
- What do you think about it now?

Remember again not to move on to analysis yet. This stage is about enabling your supervisee to consider and examine the feelings and emotions that they experienced and that possibly had an impact on the situation.

Evaluation: What was good and bad about the experience?

At this stage of the cycle you are enabling your supervisee to evaluate the event and to make value judgements. Value judgements are personal judgements or opinions based on your supervisee's ideas of what was good and bad about the experience.

Useful cue questions are:

- What was good or positive about the experience?
- What went well?
- What was bad or negative about the experience?
- What did not go well?

Analysis: What sense can you make of the situation?

At this stage you begin to break the event down into component parts which can be explored separately if need be. There may be several specific and significant parts, so each might need analysing as to what went well and what went not so well. While analysing, help your supervisee to use theory and knowledge when forming their ideas and opinions. This stage allows for more detailed questions following on from evaluation. For example, when evaluating what had not gone well, you look at and consider the reasons for this.

Useful cue questions are:

- What was your thinking behind what you did?
- What were the reasons?
- How did your actions match your beliefs?
- How did your actions match to theory and knowledge?
- What other factors influenced your decision making?
- What sense are you beginning to make of that?
- In what ways did you or others contribute to this?
- What knowledge or research should and could have informed you?
- What are your thoughts and feeling about the experience now?
- Have you made any assumptions, at the time or now?
- What overall sense do you make of the experience?

Conclusion: What else could you have done?

Having evaluated and analysed the event from a variety of angles, your supervisee has a great deal of detail on which to base their judgements and then conclusions. Ask at first what can be concluded, in a general sense, from these experiences and the analyses they have undertaken. It is important that a detailed analysis and honest exploration of all aspects of the event have been taken into consideration, otherwise valuable opportunities for learning can be missed. Remember, the purpose of reflection is to learn from an experience. It is during this stage that your supervisee is likely to develop insight into their own and others' behaviour in terms of how they contributed to the outcome of the event.

For more specific conclusions, useful cue questions are:

- What else could have been done?
- How feasible and acceptable are these alternatives?
- What can be concluded about the situation or the way of working?
- How does this compare or link to previous experience?
- What have you learnt from the experience?
- How has this changed your knowledge of or thinking about the situation?
- What are your strengths?
- What do you need to develop?
- How can you support yourself and others as a result of this?

Action plan

This stage focuses on how your supervisee would do things differently if a similar situation arose again. As well as considering what they would do differently, it is more important to look at how they will do it differently and how they will implement that plan or process of change. It can help to imagine a similar event happening again and then to make a clear plan of what to do to make it successful and effective.

Useful cue questions are:

- How will it be different?
- How will you achieve that?
- What first steps do you need to take?
- What do you need to make that happen?
- What additional knowledge and skills do you need to develop?
- How will this incident affect your future practice?
- How will you know if it has been successful?

Following the action stage the cycle is tentatively completed but suggests that, should the situation or event occur again, then that can be the focus in using the reflective cycle again.

Using reflective cycles and models together

I feel this reflective cycle is very suitable to be used in harmony with Egan's (2002) skilled helper model, which was explored in Chapter 7. For example, when goals have been put into action these can then be reflected upon and re-evaluated. More subtle personal developments may have occurred as a result of working within the skilled helper model. For example, your supervisee, through developing new understanding of their problem, has realized they need to be more assertive in team meetings. A team meeting that they recently attended can be reflected upon in supervision using Gibbs's cycle to discover whether any re-evaluation and refinement of the goal or action plan is needed.

For a reflective framework to be effective and to be used to full benefit both of you need to be committed and have a shared understanding of the process. To introduce the framework suggested here you both could have a copy of the cycle (Figure 8.1) and follow through the process together. It therefore becomes a shared understanding and experience. Or you may want to suggest to your supervisee that they choose a reflective framework, one perhaps they are familiar with, or introduce one that you feel would suit the both of you. As a supervisor, however, familiarize yourself with some of the suggested cue questions as additional prompts and for a sense of direction for the process to follow. Given time these will become second nature. You may wish to practise by using the reflective activity that follows.

Reflective activity

- Think of a recent work experience or event that you feel it would benefit you to reflect on. Something you feel you could learn from, for example something that did not go well and needs improvement.
- Using your chosen scenario work through the reflective cycle.
- Ask yourself some of the most relevant cue questions in each stage from the ones suggested.
- On completion ask yourself what have you learnt and how will you do things differently next time.
- Now ask yourself what are the benefits of reflective practice for:

  o You.
  o Your patients and clients.
  o Your colleagues.
  o Your organization and profession.

- How might you introduce reflective practice into your supervision practice?
- How will you choose a reflective cycle or framework to use?

Conclusion

This chapter has focused on reflective practice and the benefits of applying a model or framework. A question you might be asking is: How and when will I introduce this type of reflection practice during the session along with all the other issues that the supervisee may bring? The next chapter therefore will focus on developing a framework to use for the structuring a session. The next chapter will also look at evaluating clinical supervision sessions following a period of time.

Key learning points

- Being able to define the concept of reflective practice and understand the value it has for use of clinical supervision is a first step in choosing a model or framework to use.
- There are various models and frameworks of reflection to choose from. Depending on your knowledge, skills and experiences of using reflective models, you will need to decide:

  o If you are going to use one at all.
  o If you are going to use one at the appropriate opportunities to benefit your supervisee.
  o Which one you are going to choose.

- As a supervisor, the more familiar you become with the stages of a reflective model the more flexible you will become in the use of the cue questions, as they become second nature to you.
- Over time and with more experience, the skilled supervisor will become more adept in using reflective models. You will then be able to integrate these with other techniques and methods that are used to help the supervisee focus on the quality of their practice, problem solve, and learn from their experiences for the benefit of their patients and clients.

Suggested further reading

Some suggested further reading on reflection and reflective models is: Fish and Twinn (1997), Rolfe et al. (2001), Bulman and Schutz (2004), Moon (2004), Taylor (2005) and Driscoll (2007).

9

Structuring and Evaluating Clinical Supervision Sessions

Chapter outcomes

By reading this chapter, doing the reflective activities, and integrating the material into your supervision practice, you should be able to:

- Acknowledge the possible range of session content a supervisee can bring to clinical supervision.
- Develop a framework to use in supervision sessions.
- Recognize the importance of having a structure for a supervision session.
- Know about and possess some skills for the beginning phase of a session.
- Know about and possess some skills for the middle phase of a session.
- Know about and possess some skills for the closing phase of a session.
- Acknowledge and recognize the value of self-assessment for continuous learning as a supervisor.
- Use and develop a reflective cycle for learning needs as a supervisor.
- Identify some important points to discuss when evaluating supervision sessions and introduce an evaluation form.

Introduction

I will start this chapter by considering some possible areas of content that your supervisee will bring to supervision to discuss and explore. You will need to familiarize yourself with these examples to help prepare for what supervision sessions may embrace. Examples on my list will overlap during the session and certainly over time with your supervisee. Remember, the purpose of clinical supervision is that all of these examples would and should embrace the normative, formative and restorative functions of supervision that were explored in Chapter 4.

Possible session content

Work practice examples

- Workload/caseload management
- Risk management
- Clinical casework
- Updating on policy guidelines, quality of service procedures and standards
- Professional codes of conduct
- New ideas and creativity
- Personal concerns

Workplace issues examples

- Team dynamics, team relationships
- Workplace stress
- Difficult and demanding situations
- Conflict

Personal and professional development examples

- Competence and confidence in work role
- Self-awareness
- Managing stress, avoiding burnout
- Identifying learning needs and opportunities for development
- Supervising or mentoring others
- Valuing and supporting others
- Personal concerns and related work issues

Ethical issues examples

- Boundaries of confidentiality in the workplace
- Moral dilemmas

Reflective activity

- What other possible examples can you add to the list?
- What areas of session content would you feel comfortable or confident in supervising?
- What areas of session content would you not feel comfortable and confident in supervising?
- Why not?
- How might you address this?

Does a session need a framework?

Having considered a list of possible examples that are going to be brought to supervision, a question now will be, do I need a framework and structure to help me work with these? Supervision is a formal process with agreed aims, so each session requires a structure to help and enable the objectives to be met. I am using the term 'structure' to mean that you do have a sense of direction and organization during the session: that the session has a beginning, middle and end, for example. A particular framework can be used in supervision to provide structure for the exploration and reflection on the issues that the supervisee brings. There is a variety and diversity of models and frameworks to help and enable the structure, some developed specifically for clinical supervision sessions, others adapted from reflective practice and others from related theoretical perspectives. The title of a book by Eric Berne (1978) is *What Do You Say After You Say Hello?* This is a fascinating book on transactional analysis, which is about analysing transactions between people and a host of other dynamics that go on in relationships. A question you might be asking when considering how to structure a session may very well be, 'What do I do after saying hello?' Or, more probably, 'How do I start?' Some good news and some bad news, depending on your viewpoint, for the answer to that question is, 'It depends and the choice is yours.'

A danger of using frameworks is that you will concentrate too much on what the next stage is. Rather than actively listening to your supervisee, you are asking yourself, 'Am I following the stages in the correct order?' or 'What do I ask next?' You can become lost and unfocused because you are too busy concentrating on the framework. The irony here is that frameworks exist to enable you to have structure. With practice, however, you will become familiar with a framework that suits you and the needs of your supervisee.

In keeping with the spirit of supervision I will veer away from being prescriptive and advising you on what framework to employ for your session, as you will learn the most from exploring and developing that for yourself. More important when taking your first steps with clinical supervision is to model the relationship, meaning to sculpt and create a relationship that can foster the personal and professional development of the supervisee. The quality of supervision that is given and received is going to depend largely on the relationship and the unique characteristics and strengths you both bring together for the purpose of supervision. This is a human activity and a unique opportunity for you to develop wholeness and compassion in the relationship with your supervisee, in having full presence you are giving a present. Listen and learn from your supervisee, as they have rewards for you also. A first priority is to concentrate on bonding and engaging with your supervisee and creating a spirit of supervision. If you begin by concentrating too much on a framework to use, you can hinder your authenticity, empathic understanding and the quality of attention to your supervisee. I therefore feel it is unwise, at this stage, to prescribe exactly what framework to use for your session.

Which framework to choose?

What methods to use and the direction a session takes will largely be determined by the agenda the supervisee brings to the session, along with their own skills and abilities to explore and reflect. This will depend on the experience the supervisee has had of supervision in the past. If your supervisee is experienced then you will need to be flexible rather than having a prescribed framework for your sessions. If, like you, they are relatively new to supervision, then they will be looking to you to direct. I suggest you practise and experiment with various models and frameworks. You may have a preferred style developed from your own experience, knowledge and training; however, it is worth expanding your repertoire of techniques and interventions. Becoming a supervisor is an exciting opportunity for you to develop, experiment and learn. Remember, however, to always share and explain any new methods and ways of working that you are going to introduce into your sessions and ask your supervisee for feedback. Also remember that a framework needs to match your own approach, the needs of the supervisee, their workload and organization. Lynch et al. (2008: 127) rightly point out that *'it is more important to adapt the model to suit your approach than to adapt your approach to suit the model.'* This is to say that the frameworks you are using should suit you both and the needs of the session, and you should not contrive to make the session fit in with the framework.

There are an increasing number of suggested frameworks for structuring clinical supervision sessions – and note they are suggested and not prescribed. Bond and Holland (1998), Power (1999), Driscoll (2000) and Hawkins and Shohet (2000) are among several authors that focus on frameworks for supervision in healthcare settings. Lynch et al. (2008) provide an overview of several therapeutic, nursing and reflective models that are commonly used for clinical supervision suited for a variety of contexts.

Common themes to these are:

- Keep a sense of direction
- Exploration
- Focus
- Clarification
- Analysis
- Action planning
- Evaluation

Some follow the paths of reflective cycles whereas others allow for reflecting on the process and relationship between supervisee and patient and between supervisor and supervisee. There are psychodynamic models that look at unconscious processes of relationships, and solution-focused models that look at strengths to find the solutions rather than dwelling on the problem and the past. It can be confusing knowing which to choose. At first, though, it is important to develop and establish your own style, and to use what you feel comfortable with and works well with your supervisee. I suggest you familiarize yourself with different approaches that you feel competent with, so that over time and with experience you will be able to integrate various theories and frameworks into your own supervision style. I also suggest, if you are taking your first steps as a supervisor, to keep it simple. I offer here a simple format to help get you started on structuring your session. The format has a mixture of direction, flexibility and purpose.

A simple format for a session

- **Starting the session**. Welcome and settling down.
- **Beginning phase**. Setting the agenda.
- **Middle phase**. Working on the main topics and issues.
- **Closing phase**. Concluding, summarizing and evaluating.

A simple format

Starting a session: welcome and settling down

Take a few minutes to warmly welcome and help settle your supervisee, and be aware of their demeanour when they arrive. Take a mental note of remarks and comments they may make on arrival, along with significant non-verbal communication that may indicate an attitude or mood. If they appear hurried or anxious you will need to spend a little more time to help them settle into the session. With more experience you can observe important cues and clues as to the messages they are communicating to you regarding any anxieties about supervision or their general sense of well-being. If you have not done this previously, then inform your supervisee of how you like to structure the session and your style of facilitation.

Reflective activity

- How are you going to make your supervisee welcome?
- How carefully have you considered the room and environment?
- How might you help them to feel at ease, safe and relaxed?
- How do you establish and build rapport from the outset?
- How are you going to prepare yourself?
- How will you inform them of how you are to structure the session?

Beginning phase: setting the agenda

This phase of beginning the session is about setting the agenda and energizing your supervisee. Some suggestions of how this might be done are as follows.

Review and evaluate from the last session

Before you ask your supervisee what they wish to bring and what's on their agenda for the session today, briefly review and update anything that is ongoing from your last session. This will very much vary on the context of the supervisee's work. Do they have an ongoing caseload of clients, some to update you on from conclusions or action plans following your last meeting? Were there other issues raised that they need to give you feedback on? Remember, it communicates your genuineness and interest to make statements such as, 'I remember last time you were talking about . . . How did it go?' If your supervisee has an ever-changing patient group or workload then you have the opportunity to make an enquiry as to how they got on with something they were planning, a challenging situation that they were due to face or an exciting opportunity they were looking forward to. Or simply make a general enquiry by asking how things are and then ask what they want to talk about today. However, keep a mental and verbal note of themes and issues they raise, to bring a sense of progression into the sessions that you can give feedback and make comments on over time. This again communicates that you are listening and that supervision is about continuity and development, rather than one-off sessions that happen once a month.

Set today's agenda

The word 'agenda' sounds rather formal, so choose your own way of inviting the topics that the supervisee wishes to talk about. If your supervisee has come unprepared for supervision or they do not have a great deal to talk about, then use this as an opportunity to reflect on what is going well at the moment or on a professional learning need. You may, however, need to explore again what they want to use supervision for and how the time can be spent. Sensitively, and with support, remind them of their responsibility to come prepared for supervision and negotiate and explore together how they might prepare and make the most of supervision. Spend time exploring and clarifying the use of supervision to meet their professional needs, offer examples from your own practice that are relevant to help stimulate, and give constructive feedback on their strengths.

If there are several issues on the agenda then negotiate priority of order. This can be achieved through appropriate prompting and asking to say a little more about each issue. It is important to establish early in the session the main issue(s) to focus on rather than spreading time thinly over a range of broad topics, as this can result in having a general discussion with no particular direction or constructive outcome. The supervisee may feel they have cleared several items off their chest, and although you have been supportive and you have listened, ask yourself whether this valuable time has been as productive as it might and whether there has been a learning outcome.

Ask open questions

Open questions and prompting will help outline the issues. For example:

- 'What do you want to work on first?'
- 'Which of the issues you have outlined is the most urgent or important for you?'
- 'What would you like from today's session, bearing in mind all that is going on for you?'

Negotiate together the importance of topics so you can put them in order and keep in mind roughly the time you will spend on each.

Give active encouragement and energize

During the agenda setting demonstrate your enthusiasm, which will help to energize your supervisee for the session. Remember that tone of voice and body language also communicate your enthusiasm. Some examples you could use are:

- 'Yes, it seems that you have thought about that a great deal, I think that's a good place to start.'

- 'Okay, that sounds like new ground for you and well worth exploring.'
- 'Which of those do you feel will stretch you the most?'

Reflective activity

- How will you review and ask for an update of the previous session?
- How will you negotiate and agree on the agenda?
- How might you, and under what considerations will you help them to prioritize?
- How will you allocate time if there are several issues?
- How will you encourage, motivate and energize the supervisee for the session?

Middle phase: working on the main topics and issues

The middle phase is where you have a choice from among the frameworks suggested in this book and elsewhere. It will help to have a map in your mind of where to start with the presenting issues and of the direction to take. Always keep in mind the normative, formative and restorative functions as underpinning intentions when supervising. These should always be your starting objectives and aims throughout the session.

Different frameworks for use during sessions can be adapted and should be flexible. For example, appropriate stages from Egan's (2002) skilled helper model can be utilized in accordance with the issues and needs your supervisee has. The stages and skills of a problem-solving framework were explored in Chapter 7 because they are adaptable to a variety of supervision content and are fairly simplistic. Gibbs's (1998) reflective cycle was the focus of Chapter 8. This framework, with its phases and cue questions, is suitable to provide a structure when reflecting back on the supervisee's experience of practice or a situation they found themself in and wish to learn from.

To help you begin to identify with the new ideas and ways of working, here are some key words and themes to use as prompts for the session framework.

Egan's framework
- **Assessment**. Explore the issue, clarify and check for understanding, define the problem, focus on the main theme to work on.
- **Planning**. Reach a new and realistic understanding of the situation, choose from a range of possible strategies for action, and consider choice and commitment when planning implementation.
- **Implementation**. Choose the strategy for action, evaluate the possible outcomes and formulate a plan.

> (Remember, this has some similarities to the nursing process: assessment, planning, implementation, evaluation.)

Gibbs's reflective framework

- Describe what happened.
- What were you thinking and feeling?
- Evaluate what was good and bad about the experience.
- Analysis and making sense of the situation.
- Conclusions: What could have been different? What else could you have done?
- Make an action plan.
- Evaluation and what happens next.

I feel there is adequate content in the two frameworks mentioned above to help you focus, explore, analyse, help set action plans and evaluate the content that your supervisee brings to the sessions. However, you do need a structure to put that in place from the outset of the session. You need to demonstrate that you are organized and have a sense of direction for the session, which is not the same as having all the answers or being in control. Remember, this is a journey for your supervisee as well as yourself, an opportunity to learn together. You need, therefore, to let go of the controlling part of you. By letting go you will be more able to enter into the spirit of the supervision relationship.

A challenge for you will be to keep calm and not get overwhelmed or over-involved in the content of the scenarios the supervisee may bring. Resist being drawn into any dramatic situation and resist any personal enquiry for your inquisitiveness that is not to benefit your learning and understanding. You may need to ask yourself whether you are just being nosy?

Reflective activity

- Are you going to decide on a framework to use for the middle phase of the session? If yes, which one(s).
- What will be the advantages for you?
- What might be some disadvantages?
- How will you evaluate its effectiveness?

Have a look at Figure 9.1 (page 179), a reflective cycle for developing supervision competences. I have formulated this framework from the stages of the nursing process to assist learning. You may want to use this to help you reflect and develop specific aspects of a framework and means to evaluate effectiveness.

Closing phase: concluding, summarizing and evaluating

You need to keep track of the time, so have a clock or a watch easily visible to you both. Leave enough time to draw summaries and conclusions. First ask your supervisee to summarize their learning or new understandings from the session. Then offer your conclusions and relevant reflections. Do not rush this process but avoid analysing the content of the issues again. There is a danger that you can confuse your supervisee by a turnaround of thinking. By all means reflect on the session yourself afterwards and bring any relevant further thoughts to the next session. If new material does emerge in the closing phase then this can be brought to the next session, as supervision is about continuous learning.

If notes are to be recorded then agree together on session content and outcomes. This can be a useful and productive opportunity to evaluate and to offer constructive feedback. Some examples you could use to evaluate are:

- 'What has been most helpful today?'
- 'Anything less helpful, to give me something to think about?'
- 'I'm glad you chose that [mention the specific issue] today for our session, I feel it demonstrates your progress.'

The closing phase also incorporates giving constructive feedback. Use phrases such as:

- 'I think it will really benefit you if you were to practise [mention the specific learning point]. It would help you to overcome the obstacle that you have been talking about that holds you back.'
- 'Well, you have demonstrated your commitment; I think you have the skills and are ready to take on that challenge.'
- 'Well done, we have covered a lot, you've worked hard.' [Remember to finish on a positive]

Reflective activity

Take some time to reflect on your most recent supervision session. Focus on the structure and overall flow of the session. Ask yourself:

- How pleased were you with the session structure?
- How do you know this?
- How could you have structured differently and to what effect?
- What have you learnt about structuring a session?

So far in this chapter we have considered choices regarding a model to use for clinical supervision sessions and, importantly, the need to have some structure and direction to the session. I have also suggested a method of evaluation to help in your development on these aspects (Figure 9.1).

The remaining sections of the chapter look at further ways and means of evaluating your development as a supervisor and finally at the impact that supervision is having on the supervisee and their immediate healthcare setting.

Interpersonal process recall

Interpersonal process recall (IPR) was originally developed as a method by which people could reassess, and thus have more understanding of, processes that take place between themselves and others. Taking this concept further, Kagan (1980) developed a method whereby counsellors could review and indentify their interpersonal exchanges that had taken place in therapy sessions. The goals of IPR are to increase counsellor awareness of covert thoughts and feelings of both client and self, to ultimately deepen the helping relationship. This method of reviewing is aided through questioning. Research in IPR has been found useful in supervisor–supervisee relationships (Bernard 1989). It enables supervisors to learn more about their own reactions and the effects they might be having on supervisees (Scaife 2001). In most relationships, we have probably said to ourselves at times, 'if only I had said that' or 'with a bit more insight I would have said that in a different way' or 'what was really going on for me then was . . .'. IPR allows us to reflect back on an interaction and mull over what could have been said differently and some of the consequences.

IPR is being introduced here in an adapted form as a method for the supervisor to review and reflect on certain aspects of a supervision session with a supervisee.

IPR can be done after any supervision session or, in particular, after one in which you feel that the relationship with the supervisee has become rather stuck. Kagan (1980) proposes that we can become diplomatic in our interventions and hence relationships. This can be because of fear and helplessness due to past experiences of being small (as a child) in a large person's world. A combination of needing and fearing others can result in avoidance of becoming more involved, so we keep a safe distance and behave diplomatically. In supervision this can manifest as an unwillingness to become more involved with the supervisee at a certain level. Inexperienced supervisors may miss important messages from the supervisee by being too engrossed with their own thoughts and concerned to say the right thing. Thus a variety of material, the interpersonal interactions between supervisor and supervisee, can go unacknowledged.

IPR can be a valuable learning tool for inexperienced supervisors and a useful method of keeping the more experienced supervisor attuned. It provides self-evaluation and enables the supervisor to:

- Process and improve understandings of interactions and interpersonal reactions.
- Enable self-assessment of skills and qualities by reflecting on strengths and recognizing areas to develop.
- Gain information that has been unacknowledged.
- Gain insight by identifying and acknowledging anxieties, apprehensions and vulnerabilities in the interactions.
- Take personal responsibility for own behaviour that can benefit the supervisee.
- Become more attuned to the dynamics of the relationship.
- Bring about motivation to change.
- Accelerate learning and self-awareness.

(Adapted from Kagan 1980)

The most common and traditional way to perform IPR is to make a recording of a session and then play it back to someone who acts as an enquirer: they ask a combination of set open-ended questions. The recaller, who is the person undertaking the self-evaluation, responds and reflects on their own understandings and the processes that were taking place during the session. However, IPR can successfully be conducted alone, as is being suggested in the following activity.

Reflective activity

Reflect back on a recent supervision session with your supervisee. Recall significant points during the session: for example, what you felt went well and what not so well; points during the session where you felt stuck by not being sure what to say or what was really happening for your supervisee; plus any other significant points that spring to mind. Bearing those points in mind, have a look at the following list of questions. Choose at random to help you reflect back, or choose selectively the question for the specific point.

- What do you think the supervisee was trying to say at that point?
- What do you think the supervisee was feeling at this point?
- What do you wish you had said to them?
- How do you think they would have reacted if you had said that?
- What would have been the risk in saying what you wanted to say?
- Can you pick up any clues from the supervisee's non-verbal behaviour?
- What was going through your mind when the supervisee said that?
- What were you feeling at that point?
- Does that feeling have any special meaning for you?
- Was there anything that prevented you from sharing some of your thoughts and feelings?
- What did you want to happen next?

- What effect did you want to have on the supervisee?
- What do you think the supervisee wanted from you?
- What kind of person do you want the supervisee to see you as being?
- What do you think the supervisee's perceptions of you are?
- Does the supervisee remind you of anyone in your life?
- Where did you want the session to end up?

(Adapted from Kagan 1980; Bernard and Goodyear 1998; Okun 2002)

The questions are in no particular order. You may note that some refer to 'at that point', meaning a particular, verbal or non-verbal interaction during the session and are designed as such. Others could be asked to yourself at appropriate points or within the general context of the session. Alternatively, you could ask these questions as an overall experience, which may then lead you into pinpointing relevant insight and learning. Now use the following self-assessment to help determine learning needs.

Self-assessment of learning

- What have you learnt about your supervision from this exercise?
- What have you learnt about yourself?
- What insights have you gained with that particular recall?
- What insights have you gained for future supervision sessions?
- How might you develop the insights gained?
- Would there be any risk?

This is a non-threatening yet important method of self-evaluation and a means of development, insight and learning.

Self-assessment checklist for clinical supervisors

To further develop your self-assessment I will introduce you to a more comprehensive checklist taken from Hawkins and Shohet (1989) with a few minor additions. It defines some of the knowledge, skills and qualities that are necessary for the overall development of the supervisor and for effective clinical supervision. Most, although not all, of the competences have been discussed earlier in this book, some in more detail than others.

Choose one of the three columns that relate to your stage of development as a supervisor at the present time, for example novice, advanced or competent. In order to identify your learning and development needs within that stage, give yourself a grade from 1 to 10, where 1 is a strong need to develop and 10 is no need to develop.

	Knowledge	Novice	Advanced	Competent
1	A. I can define clinical supervision B. I understand the aim and purpose of clinical supervision			
2	I can explain and clarify my style of supervision			
3	I understand the formative, restorative and normative functions of clinical supervision			
4	I can describe the various types of clinical supervision, e.g. one-to-one, peer and group supervision			
5	I am clear about what clinical supervision is *not*			
6	I am clear about the boundaries of supervision			
7	I know what to include in a supervision contract			
8	I am familiar with the concepts of reflective practice			
	Qualities and skills			
9	I can negotiate a contract with a supervisee			
10	I can demonstrate the following qualities in a supervisory relationship: (a) Empathy (b) Genuineness (c) Respect (d) Trustworthiness (e) Sensitivity to the supervisee's gender, age and ethnic background (f) Sensitivity to the supervisee's professional training and knowledge (g) Tact (h) Curiosity (i) Objectivity			

	Knowledge	Novice	Advanced	Competent
11	I can achieve a balance between the formative, restorative and normative functions of clinical supervision			
12	I can use the following types of intervention: Prescriptive, Informative, Confrontative, Catalytic, Cathartic, Supportive			
13	I can both give and receive constructive feedback			
14	I can use the skills of challenging appropriately			
15	I can deal with supervisees who become upset during supervision			
16	I can make appropriate use of my own experience to help the supervisee			
17	I am willing to engage in a number of learning formats, e.g. creativity, imagination, exploration, etc.			
18	I can help the supervisee to identify the impact of their own responses to the client			
19	I can motivate the supervisee			
20	I can adhere to the boundaries of clinical supervision as agreed in the contract			
21	I can develop the skill of reflective practice in supervisees			
22	I model appropriate ethical behaviour			
23	I accept and celebrate diversity			
	Additional traits and qualities			
24	Commitment to the role of clinical supervisor			
25	Able to convey enthusiasm for clinical supervision			

	Knowledge	Novice	Advanced	Competent
26	A. Willing to negotiate B. Able to be flexible and adaptable as and when appropriate			
27	Able to bring a sense of humour			
28	A. Recognize my own strengths and limitations as a supervisor B. Courage to expose vulnerabilities, make mistakes and take risks			
29	A. Recognize my own need for clinical supervision B. Committed to updating knowledge and skills of clinical supervision			
30	Meet with other supervisors/seniors to exchange feedback and reflect on the role of clinical supervisor			

Try not to think of the self-assessment as a tall order: effective supervisors should continually reflect on their work and continue to learn throughout their career. To help you in your development as a supervisor I have formulated the reflective cycle shown in Figure 9.1 opposite. I have used the headings from the nursing process for the four stages and offered some cue questions for you to reflect on. Use the above self-assessment checklist as a guide to identify which areas of your own supervision practice you wish to develop. With a specific learning need, use the cue questions and stages in the reflective cycle (Figure 9.1) as a way forward in addressing those learning needs. This framework can be used for any number of different competences you want to develop.

Evaluation in clinical supervision

I do not intend here to evaluate clinical supervision in terms of the impact it has on clinical practice. As Bond and Holland (1998: 226) state, that is 'notoriously difficult'. However, we can assist the researchers by evaluating what goes on in clinical supervision sessions and offer both attendance records and summative evaluations to the interested stakeholders. I acknowledge this may sound daunting and stressful to both supervisee and supervisor. The rationale

Stage 1: Assessment
Identify present competences
What am I good at?
How do I know?
What do I need to develop?
How do I know?

Stage 2: Planning
How can I improve?
How do I go about it?
What skills do I have?
What resources do I have?
What skills do I need?
Who can help me?

Stage 3: Implementing
What do I do?
When will I do it?
With whom will I do it?
Who will support me?

Stage 4: Evaluation
Has there been a change?
How do I know?
What were the outcomes?
Are my findings backed up by
appropriate evidence-based literature?
Have I developed professionally?

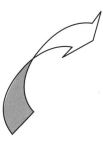
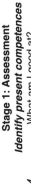
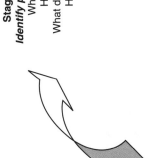
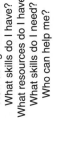
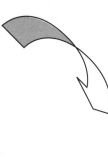
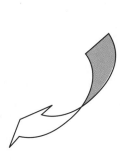
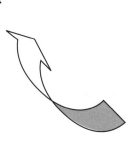
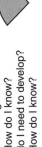

FIGURE 9.1 A reflective cycle for developing supervision competences

is not monitoring quality of care, but to give credibility to the function and purpose of supervision, and you do have a professional responsibility to give feedback and evaluation.

A supervisor's willingness to be evaluated by their supervisee clearly demonstrates commitment to all those concerned in the process and indicates that we are not asking others to do something that we are not willing to do. Bernard and Goodyear (2003) state that evaluation is fundamental and central to the supervision process. Figure 9.2 offers an example of how the supervisor and supervisee can evaluate their working relationship and the impact that

---

Name of Supervisor............................... Name of Supervisee............................

How often, e.g. monthly............................... How many sessions attended......................

1. Identify any changes that you have made have made to your clinical practice or to the way you work.

2. What evidence have you used / is there to assess or evaluate this change?

3. To whom has this change been beneficial:
   A. To you as supervisee?   **Yes / No**
   What evidence or reasons can you give?

   B. To your work colleagues and team?   **Yes / No**
   What evidence or reasons can you give?

   C. To your patients/clients with whom you work?   **Yes / No**
   What evidence or reasons can you give?

4. How will you continue to evaluate or monitor any changes to:
   A.

   B.

   C.

5. Identify any key or significant learning as a result of clinical supervision.

6. Over the past .... [no. of sessions / months] of clinical supervision:
   A. What has been the most beneficial / helpful?

   B. What has been the least beneficial / helpful?

7. What are your supervisor's / supervisee's strengths?

8. How might your supervisor / supervisee develop?

9. What changes would you like to make and discuss regarding your progress or development in clinical supervision?

10. How would you implement any of these changes?

FIGURE 9.2 Evaluation of clinical supervision sessions

supervision has on the supervisee. These evaluations, which should have been built into the contract and previously discussed, can be used on a medium-to long-term basis and also when supervision has to come to an end. It will have been important to have talked about the evaluation process at the start of the relationship and to have emphasized the positive experience for growth and learning for you both: viewing this as a joint responsibility and process can help reduce anxiety and give it positive structure and meaning.

The evaluation form offered in Figure 9.2 can be filled in by both supervisee and the supervisor, the focus is on the impact that clinical supervision has had on the supervisee's personal and professional development. The form should be given to your supervisee a session in advance, so they have time to reflect and think about the comments they are to make. I suggest you spend most, if not all, of a session on the evaluation to give it credibility and value. The supervisor will also fill out a duplicate form with their evaluations and observations on the supervisee. Both of you will then offer your thoughts, reflections and impressions to each other at the review session. Remember the guidelines for giving feedback in Chapter 3; a general principle is that the supervisee is more likely to hear and take on board any corrective feedback when this is preceded by positive feedback. The evaluation should focus on professional work, not personal issues.

When clinical supervision comes to an end

There will come a time when the sessions with your supervisee will need to come to an end. Three possible reasons for this are:

- A supervisee needs a change of supervisor for a new challenge and different experience or as a result of a change and development in their clinical skills. It is healthy to change supervisors every two to three years, so do not take this personally. They are moving on for their professional development. Think positive: you have greatly contributed.
- External or organizational reasons mean that either one of you can no longer fulfil the agreed contractual arrangements for meetings.
- Some problem or issue has arisen in the relationship that has, despite negotiation and facilitation, remained unsolved.

Plan the ending and final evaluation well in advance whenever possible. As well as the evaluation format you have used previously for your annual review, think about some completing questions for you both to talk about and share. These can take on a wider perspective to look at the supervision that has taken place between you both and to offer each other final feedback. For example:

- Have we achieved the goals we set out to achieve?
- What else have we achieved?
- What, overall, have you valued most?
- What will you miss most?
- What will you miss least?
- What have I learnt in working with you?

Conclusion

This chapter has focused on the need and value of having a structure to your sessions from the commencement of clinical supervision. Over time, and with practice, you will develop further frameworks to use while also recognizing the value of evaluation. Also over time it is important to recognize when and if you are becoming overburdened and stressed. You need to stay competent and effective in the role of clinical supervisor, so the next and last chapter will focus on ways to take care of yourself.

Key learning points

- The first-time supervisor should be aware of, and familiarize themself with, a range of subjects which may be presented in supervision.
- A skilled supervisor is aware of various frameworks that will enable them to structure the session, while also recognizing the needs of the supervisee and the overall aims and objectives of clinical supervision.
- By following a simple structure of having a beginning phase, a middle phase and a closing phase to the session, a skilled supervisor will be able to develop various methods and techniques and to integrate them into their supervision practice.
- Supervision is about continuous learning and development so a supervisor will need to be committed to self-assessing their skills and competences by reflecting on and reviewing their performance.
- Evaluation is an essential and important component of supervision and a skilled supervisor will be able to introduce this competently and successfully at the prescribed intervals.

10

Avoiding Stress and Burnout as a Supervisor

Chapter outcomes

By reading this chapter, doing the reflective activities, and integrating the material into your supervision practice, you should be able to:

- Acknowledge and recognize the difference between stress and burnout.
- Recognize and understand some warning signs and symptoms of stress.
- Recognize and understand some warning signs and symptoms of burnout.
- Acknowledge, recognize and value the importance of managing your own levels of stress.
- Know about and possess some techniques to manage your own levels of stress.
- Define and value the significance and importance of developing a spirit of supervision.
- Acknowledge and recognize the value of having supervision for your super-vision practice and identify the means by which this may be employed.

Introduction

Those of us who own a mobile phone know how often the battery needs recharging and the credit needs topping up when it is running low. I mention this to make an analogy with how often we recharge our own batteries and give ourselves credit for the work that we undertake. Just ask yourself how much work you do compared with your mobile phone. I feel it is important to consider that notion when deciding to take on an extra role to the one you already have. Especially, in the role of supervisor you have a certain responsibility to be able to contain and absorb the stresses of your supervisees while still having to manage your own levels of stress. Being a supervisor will have some level of stress which, on one hand, can be a positive stimulant and challenge for you, but, on the other hand, if it is prolonged and with little respite, can cause burnout.

Stress and burnout

There is a difference between stress and burnout. Stress in the helping professions is often caused by doing too much, having too many pressures physically and psychologically, and when there is too much demand on you and too little time. However, generally when we are stressed we can still imagine that all will be fine when things get back to normal or when we gain control again. Burnout occurs when we finally feel empty, due often to a lack of accomplishment, and there is a loss of hope for any positive change.

A certain amount of stress can be helpful; without it, for example, we would not react to situations efficiently or be stimulated to achieve the task to be carried out. A little stress, therefore, improves performance. Taking on the role of clinical supervisor will indeed raise some anxiety and stress at first, which is normal and healthy to keep you alive for the task. If these are your first steps in supervision, there is bound to be some anxiety about how you are going to perform and how you will fit supervision into your already busy workload. By staying positive and by having support, you can use a moderate amount of stress as a spur and therefore turn it to your advantage.

As a healthcare worker you need to pay attention to your levels of stress in the workplace, for if stress becomes prolonged and unrelieved there is a strong possibility that it will cause distress and lead to burnout. This will inevitably affect your performance as a supervisor. Burnout has no advantage unless it is recognized and reversed.

There is a vast amount of literature to be found on the subject of stress and burnout. My aim here is to raise awareness of the effect that prolonged stress and burnout can have, and, consequently, to emphasize that, as a clinical supervisor, it is imperative that you are aware of the signs and symptoms, for these two reasons:

- You are in a prime position as a supervisor to recognize early warning signs and levels of stress in those that you supervise.
- As a role model and competent supervisor, you need to be able to recognize early warning signs and levels in yourself.

I list below some warning signs and symptoms of stress. If they become prolonged and unless they are acknowledged and managed they can lead to the more serious condition of burnout.

Physical

- Exhaustion, feeling tired and drained most of the time
- Procrastinating, taking longer to get things done
- Headaches, back pain, aching muscles
- Lowered immunity resulting in increased vulnerability to colds and viruses
- Gastrointestinal problems
- Sleep disturbance

Behavioural

- Withdrawing from responsibilities
- Social withdrawal and isolation
- Increased absenteeism, arriving late, leaving early
- Increased alcohol or drug (licit and illicit) intake, as ways of coping
- Overeating

Emotional and psychological

- Sense of failure and self-doubt
- Negative attitudes towards self, others and life
- Constant blaming of others and building resentments to people, places and things
- Emotional distancing
- Detachment and feeling alone
- Feeling helpless, which can lead to depression
- Decreased satisfaction and sense of accomplishment
- Loss of motivation
- Beginning to feel overwhelmed by the distress or trauma of others
- Personal concerns are often intruding on the professional role

(Adapted from Helpguide.org [n.d.])

All of the above can be successfully addressed if acknowledged. It is, however, easy to slip into unconstructive ways of coping, such as overeating and increased alcohol intake. As a supervisor, you will need to aware of the constructive and healthy methods, not only to combat the symptoms but also to identify the changes that may be needed to lifestyle.

Burnout

I understand that the word 'burnout' originally alluded to unmanned space-craft: when the rocket has run out of fuel it drifts, circulates, and is of no use as it continues to burn out. The term 'burnout' in the healthcare professions is commonly used to describe the state of physical, mental and emotional exhaustion caused by excessive and prolonged stress. McLeod (2003) maintains that a state of burnout can occur when high and unrealistic aspirations of being able to provide effective help to others proves to be, for a variety of reasons, unachievable. This leaves the helper being *'unable to maintain the effort and energy required in functioning at such a high level'* (p. 428).

A first sign is probably when you begin to lose motivation and interest in the role of healthcare worker, a role that you most probably wanted and functioned well in for quite some time. I am referring here not to your role as a supervisor, but as a healthcare worker. However, if you are carrying much more than a moderate amount of stress and it is prolonged, then this surely will affect your performance as a clinical supervisor. Another sign of burnout is going through the motions and not really engaging with your clients, or even colleagues, as you generally are becoming more detached in relationships. Although you can still maintain your role of a helper, you will lose effectiveness to others and to yourself. So it is vital to be aware of this type of stress that accrues and, most importantly, to recognize and address it.

The songwriter Neil Young made a record in 1979 titled *Rust Never Sleeps*, which is a good metaphor for burnout. He was referring to the need to keep his spirit, and therefore his music, fresh and alive and not letting it corrode. As healthcare workers, we too can become rusty and corrode if we do not recognize the effects that stress can have and work on keeping ourselves and our spirit fresh and vibrant. We all have the capacity to be creative and achieve more, but we can become rusty if we do not use that ability and allow ourselves to stagnate. Ask yourself if you are keeping yourself and your spirit fresh and alive.

A first step in recognizing, and then dealing with, burnout is to be aware of some of the causes. It is difficult for many of us to admit to ourself and others that we are under stress or in danger of burnout. Indeed, we may be unable to acknowledge burnout until someone else recognizes it for us. Recognizing early warning signs is essential, as leaving them alone and avoiding taking remedies will mean the symptoms will only get worse.

By raising your own awareness of the signs and symptoms of prolonged stress and some common causes of burnout you will be better equipped to recognize them in others.

What causes burnout?

Murgatroyd (1985) noted a number of causes of burnout which healthcare workers need to be aware of and be mindful to avoid:

- Doing the same type of helping over and over again with little variation.
- Giving a great deal of one's own emotional and personal energy to others but getting little back.
- Being under constant pressure to produce results.
- Working with difficult and demanding patient and client groups.
- Receiving or hearing more criticism than support.
- Lack of trust or lack of information between those who engage in helping and those who manage the organization resources that make helping possible.
- Not having the opportunity to take new directions, to develop one's own approach or to be creative with new ways of working; being unnecessarily constrained.
- Having few opportunities for training, continuing education, supervision or support.
- Unresolved personal conflicts or problems beyond the helping work engaged in, which interfere with the helper's ability to be effective.

Reflective activity

- What other possible causes of burnout can you identify and add to the above list?
- What additional signs and symptoms of stress are you able to identify?
- What tends to stress you in your work role?
- What means and methods do you employ to relieve stress?
- How would you recognize signs or symptoms of stress in your supervisee?
- How might you help, enable and inform your supervisee in their stress management?

Taking care of yourself

Cutcliffe et al. (2001) put forward the notion that, ultimately, clinical supervision has to be concerned with benefiting service users. They go on to say that, as potential users of healthcare we all would want the best possible care for ourselves and our significant others, and that to give the best possible care, front-line healthcare staff need to be competent and healthy. I believe strongly that clinical supervision has the potential to contribute here. Engaging in your own clinical supervision, to help keep yourself competent and healthy, I feel is both a requirement and a competence of becoming a clinical supervisor. However, supervision alone is not going to keep you healthy as a supervisor. Supervision is about creating and maintaining healthy relationships.

Do you need to step back, look at yourself at times and ask, 'Do I have a healthy relationship with myself?' Carroll (2001) notes that caring for ourselves while caring and helping others too often results in imbalance, with a deficit to self. Remember the concept of the emotional bank account (Covey 1992) in Chapter 2: that you have a responsibility to ensure that you achieve a positive balance in giving and receiving. As healthcare workers and clinical supervisors, there may be a real danger that we are giving out our help and healing to others while not taking in by caring and looking after ourselves.

I mentioned in Chapter 1 the phrase used by Shohet (1985), that we teach what we most need to learn. He cited this also at a training event I attended around the same year. It was used as an expression that real growth and development are achieved by continuing to learn about ourselves and what we may teach. I feel that sentiment is more than applicable to clinical supervisors, not only to continue in your own learning but importantly to be a role model to our supervisees in ways of being and staying healthy. The next section will consider an all-encompassing way to achieve this.

The spirit of supervision

Carroll (2001) describes the essence of supervision as both functional and philosophical. He defines the functional mode as what is done in supervision; this means the tasks and the techniques along with the methods that are used to meet the purpose. The philosophy of supervision, on the other hand, is more about the meaning and value it has for you as a person; you take fully on board its ethos and spirit. I believe that to fully value the philosophy of supervision you need to be in the spirit of supervision. Being in and having a spirit of supervision means that supervision is not just a hobby or pastime, but that there is both a will and commitment. The philosophy of supervision is enduring, becomes a style of being and is all-encompassing; it is therefore not restricted to the room where supervision occurs. Like Rogers (1980) who considered the core conditions as a way of being, and Miller and Rollnick (2002) who talk about the spirit of motivational interviewing, I believe that supervision shares comparable notions. I propose that to develop and maintain a spirit of supervision you need to:

- Value yourself.
- Value others.
- Have a real interest in people.
- Develop and maintain self-integrity.
- Radiate a positive attitude.
- Model behaviour that you wish in others.

- Admit to mistakes, be forgiving of self and others, and look for learning experiences.
- Value humour and use to uplift, energize and maintain a sense of perspective, but not at the expense of others.
- Keep in the solution and not in the problem. I have heard this sentiment expressed as feed the solution and starve the problem.
- Be open to change while not letting go of your values.
- Value lifelong learning.
- Have belief in the other's capacity to grow and develop.
- Motivate others and promote creativity and curiosity.
- Form collaborative relationships, not controlling or competitive relationships.
- Maintain healthy and prosperous relationships.
- Listen with all your senses as well as your heart, and learn.

Thus a spirit of supervision merges into the philosophy and integrates into the many different aspects of our professional relationships and in the role we have as a helper. We may, and can, also carry these principles into all our affairs.

Some ways to combat stress and replenish yourself

Here are some suggestions of ways to keep a healthy mind and spirit for the task in hand:

- Start the day with a quiet moment or thought. Or make sure you are able to have some time and space during the day to relax and have quiet time alone. Meditation is a good way to ground yourself and to gather your thoughts.
- Make a gratitude list. Gratitude is about the appreciation of people, places and things, and it is about ideas, qualities and feelings. It is also always and absolutely free. We often take many precious aspects of our lives for granted, so for attitude get gratitude. I find this a good way to let go of resentments that begin to fester.
- Vary your work as much as possible and nurture your creative side. Develop a range of interests away from work.
- Nurture friendships and relationships. One way to do this is to pay someone a compliment every day. Be specific as to what they did or said and why you appreciated it. Include your feelings, as these add strength and give more personal meaning. Another way is to hold one focused meaningful conversation with a good friend or family member each day.
- Practise acts of random kindness. Throughout the day there will be many opportunities to practise acts of kindness. A kind word, gesture or a good

deed. The rewards of self-satisfaction and a quiet joy can be yours. Doing someone a good turn when not getting found out can have greater rewards.
- Set boundaries, learn to say no to requests on your time and when inappropriate.
- Take a break from multitasking and concentrate on one thing at a time.
- Take care of your physical health. Adopt healthy eating, exercising and sleeping habits.

I mention above only a few of the ways to stay healthy and positive while combating stress. Perhaps some may not be the conventional or traditional ways of avoiding stress, but my aim is to keep within the spirit of supervision and a sense of perspective. I personally believe that being in the role of a clinical supervisor we are in a privileged position. I need to remind myself of that at various times so I do not get complacent. I find some of the above give me self-satisfaction in a constructive, creative and positive way. In essence we reap what we sow. Add to the above list your own creative ways of staying healthy in mind and spirit. You may view them to use in the context of your professional role and while at work, or, as I have already suggested, you may want to carry these principles into all aspects of your life.

Who supervises the supervisor?

Being a clinical supervisor can provide a great deal of additional job satisfaction; it will, however, require extra commitment and draw on extra of your resources. As a supervisor, you will be providing considerable emotional support for your supervisee and take on board issues that cause concern and require reflection. It is therefore essential, keeping within the principles and ethos of supervision, that you are able to receive supervision for your supervision.

A question often asked when training supervisors is, who supervises the supervisor? Page and Wosket (1994) use the analogy of parent and grandparent when addressing the above question and when the continuous line of supervision ceases. The supervisor can be said to be acting as a parent figure to the supervisee; the supervisor of the supervisor can then be said to be a grandparent figure. A supervisor new to the role will need fostering for some time while they become more effective and competent in that role. This supervisor of the supervisor (grandparent figure) can eventually withdraw as they place more trust in their supervisors. However, they are still in the background for times when the supervisor (parent) needs a reassuring figure, and the two may still meet up occasionally. You may be asking who supervises the supervisor of the supervisor. Well, the chain has now ceased, the senior supervisor (grandparent) will ensure they have contact with others in a similar role where they can meet up for mutual support.

I appreciate that within the context of many healthcare settings the arrangements for providing support for supervisors will inevitably vary and in some cases provision cannot be made at all because of the pressure on time and resources. However, there are several, more informal ways that can be employed to good effect:

- Identify and locate a peer supervisor whom you can meet up with and share equal time supervising each other. This allows you both time and space to offload any emotional issues and the concerns and anxieties that arise from your supervision practice.
- Ask your own clinical supervisor if you can utilize some of the time you spend with them, as and when needs be, to reflect on your supervision as well as your clinical practice.
- When and if you take on three or more supervisees I would suggest forming a peer group with other similar supervisors. This format of group supervision for supervisors has all the benefits of peer supervision (as above) but can also provide additional support, challenge and learning from each other. This may also be an opportunity to develop group supervision skills with your peers for later use if you are to become a group supervisor.

Conclusion

As we are coming to the end of this book on first steps in clinical supervision you may feel there is much to take on board and learn. I am reminded at this point of the term 'psychological furniture', which is a phrase used to symbolize the taking in (psychologically) of new concepts (furniture) and accommodating them alongside those you already have. I often use this term at the end of a training day or when there is some confusion regarding learning new material on a particular subject of a mental nature. Picture in your mind the concept of clinical supervision and imagine this as a house. The psychological furniture that is stored there is what you currently own and understand regarding the concept of clinical supervision. These pieces of furniture represent your current ideas, beliefs, techniques, skills and so on. You are now being asked, through reading this book, to consider and accommodate some new ideas, values, beliefs, techniques, skills and so on. So, what do you do with all this psychological furniture? It no doubt calls for some rearranging, and the questions you may have are:

- Will this new furniture fit alongside what you already have?
- Is there enough room?
- Does it match your colour scheme?

- Does this mean you need to throw out of some of the old furniture?
- How comfortable are you with the new furniture?

Taking on the role of clinical supervisor may feel like this at first, as you are bringing in and developing new ideas while letting go of some of the old ones that have served you well. Quite possibly you may feel uncertain at first. Remember some of the principles about clinical supervision that you have read about to help you. Reflect, and share with appropriate others, your thoughts and ideas about developing your supervision practice. Ask for open and honest feedback on your learning and development. Supervisors are not perfect and do not have all the answers, but remember that supervision is lifelong learning and that we are still developing and seeking progress. So, may your practice as a clinical supervisor bring out the best in you, while at the same time, bring out the best in those that you supervise.

Key learning points

- A moderate amount of stress can help stimulate and enable a person to achieve, but prolonged stress, unless recognized and relieved, is unhealthy and can cause burnout.
- As a supervisor, you are in a key position to help acknowledge and recognize stress in those you are working with.
- You therefore have a responsibility to constantly monitor your own levels of stress in order to be effective as a supervisor and to be a competent role model.
- Ensure you have the right amount of support and supervision for your own practice as a healthcare worker and for your role as clinical supervisor.
- By being creative and constructive in the ways and means of relieving stress you are also able to use these principles to benefit all aspects of your well-being.
- Aim to develop and create the spirit of supervision as you progress in your development as a clinical supervisor and health care worker.

References

Argyle, M. (1975) *Bodily Communication*. London: Methuen.

Argyle, M. (1994) *The Psychology of Interpersonal Behaviour*, 5th edn. London: Penguin.

Ashmore, R. (1999) Heron's Intervention Framework: an introduction and critique, *Mental Health Nursing*, 19(1): 24–7.

Berger, S.S. and Buchholz, E.S. (1993) On becoming a supervisee: preparation for learning in a supervisory relationship. *Psychotherapy*, 30(1): 1–9.

Bernard, J.M. (1989) Training supervisors to examine relationships issues using IPR. *The Clinical Supervisor*, 7: 103–12.

Bernard, J.M. and Goodyear, R.K. (1998) *Fundamentals of Clinical Supervision*, 2nd edn. Needham Heights: Allyn & Bacon.

Bernard, J.M. and Goodyear, R.K. (2003) *Fundamentals of Clinical Supervision*, 3rd edn. Boston: Allyn & Bacon.

Berne, E. (1978) *What Do You Say After You Say Hello?* New York: Grove Press.

Bond, M. and Holland, S. (1998) *Skills of Clinical Supervision for Nurses*. Buckingham: Open University Press.

Borders, L.D. (2005) Snapshot of clinical supervision in counseling and counselor education: a five-year review, *Supervision in Counseling: Interdisciplinary Issues and Research*, 24: 49–67.

Boud, D., Keogh, R. and Walker, D. (1985) *Reflection: Turning Experience into Learning*. London: Kogan Page.

Boyd, E. and Fales, A. (1983) Reflective learning: the key to learning from experience, *Journal of Humanistic Psychology*, 23(2): 99–117.

Brocklehurst, N. (1994) Developing a model of supervision for community nursing. Unpublished MSc thesis, University of Manchester.

Brown, A. and Bourne, I. (1996) *The Social Work Supervisor*. Buckingham: Open University Press.

Bulman, C. and Schutz, S. (eds) (2004) *Reflective Practice in Nursing*, 3rd edn. Oxford: Blackwell.

Burgoon, J., Buller, D. and Woodall W.G. (1996) *Nonverbal Communication: The Unspoken Dialogue*, 2nd edn. New York: McGraw-Hill.

Burnard, P. (1985) *Learning Human Skills: A Guide for Nurses*. London: Heinemann.

Burnard, P. (1992) *Know Yourself! Self-awareness Activities for Nurses*. London: Scutari Press.

Burnard, P. (1998) Listening as a personal quality, *Journal of Community Nursing*, 12(2): 32–4.

Burnard, P. and Morrison, P. (1988) Nurses' perceptions of their interpersonal skills: a descriptive study using Six Category Intervention Analysis, *Nurse Education Today*, 8: 266–72.

Butterworth, A. and Faugier, J. (eds) (1992) *Clinical Supervision and Mentorship in Nursing*. London: Chapman & Hall.

Butterworth, A., Carson, J., White, E., Jeacock, J. and Clements, A. (1997) *It's Good To Talk?* University of Manchester.

Cameron, H. (2008) *The Counselling Interview.* Houndmills: Palgrave Macmillan.

Campbell, J. (2006) *Essentials of Clinical Supervision.* Hoboken, NJ: Wiley.

Carkhuff, R.R. (1983) *The Art of Helping: Student Workbook,* 2nd edn. Amherst, MA: Human Resources Press.

Carroll, M. (2001) *Counselling Supervision: Theory, Skills and Practice (Counsellor Trainer and Supervisor).* London: Sage.

Conner, M. (1994) *Training the Counsellor.* London: Routledge.

Covey, S. (1992) *The Seven Habits of Highly Effective People.* London: Simon & Schuster.

Cutcliffe, J.R. (2000) To record or not to record: documentation in clinical supervision, *British Journal of Nursing,* 19(6): 350–5.

Cutcliffe, J.R. (2001) Personal, professional and practice development, in J.R. Cutcliffe, T. Butterworth and B. Proctor (eds), *Fundamental Themes in Clinical Supervision.* London: Routledge.

Cutcliffe, J.R. and Epling, M. (1997) An exploration of the use of John Heron's confronting interventions in clinical supervision: case studies from practice, *Psychiatric Care,* 44: 174–80.

Cutcliffe, J.R., Butterworth, T. and Proctor, B. (eds) (2001) *Fundamental Themes in Clinical Supervision.* London: Routledge.

Daloz, L. (1986) *Effective Teaching and Mentoring.* London: Jossey-Bass.

De Bono, E. (1992) *Serious Creativity: Using the Power of Lateral Thinking to Create New Ideas.* New York: Harper Business.

Department of Health (1993) *Vision for the Future: The Nursing, Midwifery and Health Visiting Contribution to Health and Health Care.* London: HMSO.

Diamond, B. (1998a) Legal aspects of clinical supervision 1: employer vs employee, *British Journal of Nursing,* 7(7): 393–5.

Diamond, B. (1998b) Legal aspects of clinical supervision 2: professional accountability, *British Journal of Nursing,* 7(8): 487–9.

Driscoll, J. (2000) *Practising Clinical Supervision: A Reflective Approach.* London: Baillière Tindall.

Driscoll, J. (2007) *Practising Clinical Supervision: A Reflective Approach for Healthcare Professionals,* 2nd edn. London: Baillière Tindall.

Egan, G. (1985) *Exercises in Helping Skills: A Manual to Accompany the Skilled Helper,* 3rd edn. Pacific Grove, CA: Brooks/Cole.

Egan, G. (2002) *The Skilled Helper,* 7th edn. Pacific Grove, CA: Brooks/Cole.

Faugier, J. (1992) The supervision relationship, in A. Butterworth and J. Faugier (eds), *Clinical Supervision and Mentorship in Nursing.* London: Chapman & Hall.

Faugier, J. (1996) Clinical supervision and mental health nursing, in T. Sandford and K. Gourney (eds), *Perspectives in Mental Health Nursing.* London: Chapman & Hall.

Fish, D. and Twinn, S. (1997) *Quality Clinical Supervision in the Health Care Professions: Principled Approaches to Practice.* Oxford: Butterworth-Heinemann.

Fisher, M. (1996) Using reflective practice in clinical supervision, *Professional Nurse,* 11(7): 443–4.

Fitzgerald, M. (2000) Clinical supervision and reflective practice, in C. Bulman and S. Burns (eds), *Reflective Practice in Nursing,* 2nd edn. Oxford: Blackwell.

Fowler, J. (1996) The organisation of clinical supervision within the nursing profession, *Journal of Advanced Nursing,* 23: 471–8.

Fowler, J. (2007) Using solution-focused techniques in clinical supervision, *Nursing Times*, 13(22): 30–1.

Frankland, A. and Sanders, P. (1995) *Next Steps in Counselling*. Manchester: PCCS Books.

Freshwater, D. (2003) *Counselling Skills for Nurses, Midwives and Health Visitors*. Maidenhead: Open University Press.

Gibbs, G. (1988) *Learning by Doing: Guide to Teaching and Learning Methods*. Further Education Unit, Oxford Polytechnic.

Gillings, B. (2000) Clinical supervision in reflective practice, in S. Burns and C. Bulman, *Reflective Practice in Nursing*. Oxford: Blackwell.

Gilmore, S. (1973) *The Counsellor in Training*. Englewood Cliffs, NJ: Prentice Hall.

Gilmore, A. (2001) Clinical supervision in nursing and health visiting, in J.R. Cutcliffe, T. Butterworth and B. Proctor (eds), *Fundamental Themes in Clinical Supervision*. London: Routledge.

Gopee, N. (2008) *Mentorship and Supervision in Healthcare*. London: Sage.

Gordon, T. (1977) *Leader Effective Training*. New York: Bantam Books.

Harvey, D.R. and Schramski, T.G. (1984) Effective supervision and consultation: a model for the development of functional supervision and consultation programmes, *Counselor Education and Supervision*, 23: 197–204.

Hawkins, P. and Shohet, R. (1989) *Supervision in the Helping Professions*. Milton Keynes: Open University Press.

Hawkins, P. and Shohet, R. (2000) *Supervision in the Helping Professions*, 2nd edn. Milton Keynes: Open University Press.

Hay, J. (2007) *Reflective Practice and Supervision for Coaches*. Maidenhead: Open University Press.

Helpguide.org (n.d.) Preventing burnout: signs symptoms, causes and oping strategies. http://helpguide.org/mental/burnout_signs_symptoms.htm (accessed 3 November 2009).

Heron, J. (1975) *Six Category Intervention Analysis*. Guildford: University of Surrey.

Heron, J. (2001) *Helping the Client: A Creative Practical Guide*, 5th edn. London: Sage.

Hewitt, J., Coffey, M. and Rooney, G. (2009) Forming, sustaining and ending therapeutic relationships, in P. Callaghan, J. Playle and L. Cooper (eds), *Mental Health Nursing Skills*. Oxford: Oxford University Press.

Hewson, J. (1999) Training supervisors to contract in supervision, in E.L. Holloway and M. Caroll (eds), *Training Counselling Supervisors*. London: Sage.

Hughes, L. and Pengelly, P. (1997) *Staff Supervision in a Turbulent Environment: Managing Process and Task in Front-Line Services*. London: Jessica Kingsley.

Inskipp, F. (1996) *Skills Training for Counselling*. London: Sage.

Inskipp, F. and Proctor, B. (1993) *The Art, Craft and Tasks of Counselling Supervision. Part 1: Making the Most of Supervision*. Twickenham: Cascade Publications.

Inskipp, F. and Proctor, B. (1995) *The Art, Craft and Tasks of Counselling Supervision. Part 2: Becoming a Supervisor*. Twickenham: Cascade Publications.

Jasper, M. (2006) *Professional Development, Reflection and Decision-Making*. Oxford: Blackwell.

Johns, C. (2004) *Becoming a Reflective Practitioner*, 2nd edn. Oxford: Blackwell.

Kadushin, A. (1992) *Supervision in Social Work*, 3rd edn. New York: Columbia University Press.

Kagan, N. (1980) Influencing human interaction – eighteen years with IPR, in A.K. Hess (ed.), *Psychotherapy Supervision: Theory, Research, and Practice*. New York: Wiley.

Kavanagh, D.J., Spence, S.H., Wilson, J. and Crow, N. (2002) Achieving effective supervision, *Drug and Alcohol Review*, 21: 247–52.

Kilminster, S.M. and Jolly, B.C. (2000) Effective supervision in clinical practice settings: a review of the literature, *Medical Education*, 34(10): 827–40.

King's Fund Centre (1994) *Clinical Supervision in Practice*. London: King's Fund Centre.

Knapp, M.L. (1978) *Non-verbal Communication in Human Interaction*. New York: Rinehart & Winstson.

Knowles, M. (1984) *The Adult Learner: A Neglected Species*. Houston, TX: Gulf Publishing.

Kohner, N. (1994) *Clinical Supervision in Practice*. London: King's Fund Centre.

Kottkamp, R. (1990) Means of facilitating reflection, *Education and Urban Society*, 22(2): 182–203.

Lewis, R.D. (2008) *Cross-cultural Communication: A Visual Approach*, 2nd edn. Winchester: Transcreen Publications.

Luft, J. (1969) *Of Human Interaction*. Palo Alto, CA: Mayfield Publishing.

Lynch, L., Hancox, K., Happle, B. and Parker, J. (2008) *Clinical Supervision for Nurses*. Chichester: Wiley–Blackwell.

Martin, S. (1996) Support and challenge: conflicting or complementary aspects of mentoring novice teachers? *Teachers and Teaching: Theory and Practice*, 2(1): 41–56

Maslow, A. (1987) *Motivation and Personality*, 3rd edn. New York: Harper & Row.

McCabe, C. and Timmins, F. (2006) *Communication Skills for Nursing Practice*. Houndmills: Palgrave Macmillan.

McLeod, J. (2003) *An Introduction to Counselling*, 3rd edn. Maidenhead: Open University Press.

McLeod, J. (2007) *Counselling Skill*. Maidenhead: Open University Press.

McNally, J., Cope, P., Inglis, B. and Stronach, I. (1997) The student teacher in school; conditions for development, *Teaching and Teacher Education*, 13(5): 485–98

Miller, W.R. and Rollnick, S. (2002) *Motivational Interviewing: Preparing People for Change*. New York: Guilford Press.

Milne, D. and Westerman, C. (2001) Evidence-based clinical supervision: rationale and illustration *Clinical Psychology and Psychotherapy*, 8: 444–57.

Moon, J. (2004) *A Handbook of Reflective and Experiential Practice*. Abingdon: Routledge.

Morris, D. (1994) *Bodytalk: The Meaning of Human Gestures*. New York: Crown Trade Paperbacks.

Morrison, P. and Burnard, P. (1998) *Caring and Communicating: The Interpersonal Relationship in Nursing*. London: Palgrave Macmillan.

Morrissey, J. (2009) Interpersonal communication: Heron's Six Category Intervention Analysis, in P. Callaghan, J. Playle and L. Cooper (eds), *Mental Health Nursing Skills*. Oxford: Oxford University Press.

Morse, J.M. (1991) Negotiating commitment and involvement in the nurse–patient relationship, *Journal of Advanced Nursing*, 16: 455–68.

Murgatroyd, S. (1985) *Counselling and Helping*. London: Methuen.

Nelson-Jones, R. (2008) *Basic Counselling Skill: A Helper's Manual*. London: Sage.

Nicholls, D. (2007) Essential elements for a successful supervisory partnership to flourish, in J. Driscoll (ed.), *Practising Clinical Supervision*, 2nd edn. Edinburgh: Baillière Tindall.

Nursing and Midwifery Council (2005) Supporting Nurses and Midwives through Lifelong Learning. London: NMC.

Nursing and Midwifery Council (2008) The Code – Standards of Conduct, Performance and Ethics to Nurses and Midwives. London: NMC.

Okun, B. (2002) *Effective Helping*, 6th edn. Pacific Grove, CA: Brookes/Cole.

Palmer, A.M., Burns, S. and Bulman, C. (1994) *Reflective Practice in Nursing: The Growth of the Professional Practitioner*. Oxford: Blackwell.

Page, S. and Wosket, V. (1994) *Supervising the Counsellor*. London: Routledge.

Pendleton, D., Schofield, T., Tate, P. and Havelock, P. (1984) *The Consultation: An Approach to Learning and Teaching*. Oxford: Oxford University Press.

Platzer, H., Snelling, J. and Blake, D. (1997) Promoting reflective practitioners in nursing, *Teaching In Higher Education*, 2: 103–21.

Powell, D.J. (2004) *Clinical Supervision in Alcohol and Drug Abuse Counselling*. San Francisco: Jossey-Bass.

Power, S. (1999) *Nursing Supervision: A Guide for Clinical Practice*. London: Sage.

Proctor, B. (1986) Supervision: a co-operative exercise in accountability, in M. Marken and M. Payne (eds), *Enabling and Ensuring*. National Youth Bureau and Council for Education and Training in Youth and Community Work, Leicester.

Proctor, B. (1991) On being a trainer, in W. Dryden and B. Thorene (eds), *Training and Supervision for Counselling in Action*. London: Sage.

Proctor, B. (2008) *Group Supervision: A Guide to Creative Practice*, 2nd edn. London: Sage.

Rafferty, M., Llewellyn-Davies, B. and Hewitt, J. (2007) Setting standards for the practice of clinical supervision: a Welsh perspective, in J. Driscoll (ed.), *Practising Clinical Supervision: A Reflective Approach for Healthcare Professionals*, 2nd edn. Edinburgh: Baillière Tindall.

Rogers, C. (1957) The necessary and sufficient conditions of therapeutic personality change, *Journal of Consulting Psychology*, 21: 95–103.

Rogers, C. (1961) *On Becoming a Person*. London: Constable.

Rogers, C. (1969) *Freedom to Learn*. Columbus, OH: Merrill.

Rogers, C. (1980) *A Way of Being*. Boston, MA: Houghton Mifflin.

Rogers, C. (1983) *Freedom to Learn for the 80s*. Columbus, OH: Merrill.

Rogers, J. (2004) *Coaching Skills: A Handbook*. Maidenhead: Open University Press

Rolfe, G., Freshwater, D. and Jasper, M. (2001) *Critical Reflection for Nursing and the Helping Professions: A User's Guide*. London: Palgrave Macmillan.

Rungapadiachy, D.M. (1999) *Interpersonal Communication and Psychology for Health Care Professionals: Theory and Practice*. Oxford: Butterworth–Heinemann.

Sanders, P. (1994) *First Steps in Counselling*. Manchester: PCCS Books.

Sanders, P., Frankland, A. and Wilkins, P. (2009) *Next Steps in Counselling Practice*. Ross-on-Wye: PCCS Books.

Scaife, J. (2001) *Supervision in the Mental Health Professions*. London: Brunner–Routledge.

Scaife, J. (2009) *Supervision in Clinical Practice: A Practitioner's Guide*. London: Routledge.

Schön, D. (1983) *The Reflective Practitioner*. London: Temple Smith.

Shohet, R. (1985) *Dreamsharing*. Wellingborough: Turnstone Press.

Shohet, R. (2008) *Passionate Supervision*. London: Jessica Kingsley.

Simms, J. (1993) In G. Swain (1995) *Clinical Supervision: The Principles and Process*. London: College Hill Press.

Sloan, G. and Watson, H. (2002) Clinical supervision models for nursing: structure research and limitations, *Nursing Standard*, 17(4): 41–6.

Stein-Parbury, J. (1993) *Patient and Person: Developing Interpersonal Skills in Nursing*. Melbourne: Churchill Livingstone.

Stickley, T. and Stacey, G. (2009) Caring: the essence of mental health nursing, in P. Callaghan, J. Playle and L. Cooper (eds), *Mental Health Nursing Skills*. Oxford: Oxford University Press.

Taylor, B. (2005) *Reflective Practice: A Guide for Nurses and Midwives*, 2nd edn. Buckingham: Open University Press.

Teasdale, K., Brocklehurst, N., Thom, N. et al. (2001) Clinical supervision and support for nurses: an evaluation study, *Journal of Advanced Nursing*, 33(2): 216–24.

Thompson, N. (2002) *People Skills*, 2nd edn. Houndmills: Palgrave Macmillan.

UKCC (1996) *Position Statement on Clinical Supervision for Nursing and Health Visiting*. London: UKCC.

Watkins, P. (2001) *Mental Health Nursing: The Art of Compassionate Care*. Oxford: Butterworth-Heinemann.

Webb, B. (1997) Auditing a clinical nurse training programme, *Nursing Standard*, 11: 34–9.

Wilson, T. (2000) Learning relationships: mentorship, preceptorship and clinical supervision, in P. Nicklin and N. Kenworthy (eds), *Teaching and Assessing in Nursing Practice*. Edinburgh: Baillière Tindall.

Winstanley, J. (2001) Developing methods for evaluating clinical supervision, in J.R. Cutcliffe, T. Butterworth and B. Proctor (eds), *Fundamental Themes in Clinical Supervision*. London: Routledge.

Winstanley, J. (2003) Clinical supervision: models, measures and best practice, *Nurse Research*, 10(4): 7–38.

Wosket, V. (2006) *Egan's Skilled Helper Model*. London: Routledge.

Young, N. (1979) *Rust Never Sleeps*. Reprise Records.

Index

acceptance, supervision relationship, 52–3
action strategies, problem-solving framework, 145–9
agenda, clinical supervision sessions, 168–70
agenda for change, problem-solving framework, 142–4
authority and power, 16–18

background information, 5–6
background, this supervisor's, 6–7
benefits
    clinical supervision, 13–14
    reflective practice, 155
burnout
    avoiding, 183–92
    causes, 186–7

catalytic category, six-category intervention analysis, 109, 120–1
cathartic category, six-category intervention analysis, 109, 118–20
challenge/support balance, clinical supervision, 79–82
changing supervisors, clinical supervision, 82–3
classifying clinical supervision, 10–13
clinical supervision
    see also supervision
    benefits, 13–14
    challenge/support balance, 79–82
    changing supervisors, 82–3
    classifying, 10–13
    conceptual framework, 67–9
    defining, 3–5
    formative function, 11–12, 14, 16, 72–4
    functions, 10–13, 67–84

guidelines for introducing, 19
introducing, 19
name of, 7–8
normative function, 11, 13–14, 15, 70–2
reasons for becoming a supervisor, 15–19
reflective practice, 154–5
restorative function, 12, 14, 17, 74–9
similar roles, 2–3
support/challenge balance, 79–82
target, 5–6
training, 21–2
vignette, supervision functions, 77–8
clinical supervision sessions
    agenda, 168–70
    ending, 181–2
    evaluating, 178–81
    format, 167–73
    frameworks, 165–73
    interpersonal process recall (IPR), 173–5
    self-assessment checklist, 175–8
    structuring, 163–82
closed questions, listening skills, 94–5
collaboration, supervision, 19–21
commitment, problem-solving framework, 144–5
communication
    listening skills, 89–94
    non-verbal communication, 89–94
    supervision relationship, 55
conceptual framework, clinical supervision, 67–9
confronting category, six-category intervention analysis, 109, 115–18
contracting for supervision, 36
contracts
    examples, 40–3

introducing, 40–3
making, 40–3
supervision, 40–3
core conditions, supervision
    relationship, 49–55
counselling, supervision, 9
creativity, problem-solving framework,
    140–2

degenerative interventions, six-
    category intervention analysis,
    125, 126–8
developing personal qualities,
    supervision relationship, 54–5

empathic relationship, listening skills,
    87
empathy, supervision relationship,
    49–51
evaluating clinical supervision sessions,
    178–81
expectations, supervision, 33–5

feedback, constructive, supervision
    relationship, 61–5
feeling words, restorative function,
    75–7
first meeting, 24–44
focusing, problem-solving framework,
    139–40
force-field analysis, problem-solving
    framework, 147–8
format, clinical supervision sessions,
    167–73
formative function, clinical
    supervision, 11–12, 14, 16, 72–4
frameworks
    see also problem-solving framework
    clinical supervision sessions,
    165–73
frequency, supervision, 36
functions, clinical supervision, 10–13,
    67–84
    listening skills, 87
    research, 83–4
    vignette, 77–8

genuineness, supervision relationship,
    51–2

guidelines for introducing clinical
    supervision, 19

informative category, six-category
    intervention analysis, 109, 113–14
interpersonal process recall (IPR),
    clinical supervision sessions, 173–5
intervention analysis see six-category
    intervention analysis
IPR see interpersonal process recall

Johari Window, self-awareness, 57–60

legal issues, supervision, 37
listening skills, 85–105
    closed questions, 94–5
    communication, 89–94
    core principles, 88
    empathic relationship, 87
    non-verbal communication, 89–94
    open questions, 95
    paraphrasing, 98–102
    questions, 94–6
    readiness to listen, 94
    reflecting, 98–102
    self-disclosure, 102–4
    silence, 96–8
    summarizing, 104–5
    supervision functions, 87
    as a supervisor, 86–7
    toolbox, 94–105
    understanding, 102
    'why' questions, 95–6
location, supervision, 36

model of reflection, reflective practice,
    156–60

non-verbal communication
    combining with spoken word, 91–2
    listening skills, 89–94
    perceiving, 92–4
normative function, clinical
    supervision, 11, 13–14, 15, 70–2
note taking, supervision, 37–9

open questions, listening skills, 95

paraphrasing, listening skills, 98–102

person-centred theory, supervision
   relationship, 48
power and authority, 16–18
practicalities, supervision, 36
prescriptive category, six-category
   intervention analysis, 109,
   110–12
problem-solving framework, 129–51
   action plan, 148–9
   action strategies, 145–9
   agenda for change, 142–4
   best-fit action, 146–8
   clarifying blind spots, 136–8
   commitment, 144–5
   costs and benefits, 144–5
   creativity, 140–2
   current scenario, 131–40
   focusing, 139–40
   force-field analysis, 147–8
   implementation, 148–9
   preferred scenario, 140–5
   problem situation, 131–40
   purposes, 131–3
   reality testing, 142–4
   reasons for, 131–3
   stage 1: current scenario, 131–40
   stage 2: preferred scenario, 140–5
   stage 3: action strategies, 145–9
   stages overview, 131–3

questions
   closed questions, 94–5
   listening skills, 94–6
   open questions, 95
   'why' questions, 95–6

reality testing, problem-solving
   framework, 142–4
reasons for becoming a supervisor,
   15–19
record keeping, supervision, 37–9
reflecting, listening skills, 98–102
reflective practice, 152–62
   benefits, 155
   clinical supervision, 154–5
   defining, 153–4
   model of reflection, 156–60
   reasons for, 156
reflective cycle, 156–61

relationship, supervision see
   supervision relationship
research, functions, clinical
   supervision, 83–4
responsibilities and rights, supervision
   contract, 26–9
restorative function
   clinical supervision, 12, 14, 17, 74–9
   feeling words, 75–7
rights and responsibilities, supervision
   contract, 26–9

self-assessment checklist, clinical
   supervision sessions, 175–8
self-awareness
   clinical supervisor, 55–7
   framework, 57–60
   Johari Window, 57–60
   reasons for, 55–7
   supervision relationship, 55–60
self-disclosure, listening skills, 102–4
sessions, clinical supervision see clinical
   supervision sessions
silence, listening skills, 96–8
six-category intervention analysis,
   106–28
   catalytic category, 109, 120–1
   cathartic category, 109, 118–20
   for clinical supervision, 123–6
   confronting category, 109, 115–18
   degenerative interventions, 125,
      126–8
   informative category, 109, 113–14
   interdependence, 123–6
   prescriptive category, 109, 110–12
   supportive category, 109, 121–3
   valid interventions, 124–5
   value of, 107–10
skilled helper model see problem-
   solving framework
skills, transferable, 15–17
spirit of supervision, stress, 188–9
stress
   avoiding, 183–92
   combating, 189–90
   spirit of supervision, 188–9
   supervising the supervisor, 190–1
   taking care of yourself, 187–8
   warning signs, 184–5

structuring clinical supervision
    sessions, 163–82
summarizing, listening skills, 104–5
supervising the supervisor, stress, 190–1
supervision
    see also clinical supervision
    collaboration, 19–21
    contracting for, 36
    contracts, 40–3
    counselling, 9
    defining, 3–5
    expectations, 33–5
    frequency, 36
    as a journey, 8
    legal issues, 37
    location, 36
    note taking, 37–9
    practicalities, 36
    record keeping, 37–9
    therapy, 8–10
supervision contract
    elements, 26
    purpose, 25
    responsibilities and rights, 26–9
    rights and responsibilities, 26–9
supervision relationship, 45–66
    acceptance, 52–3
    characteristics, 47–8
    communication, 55
    contributing to, 29–31
    core conditions, 49–55

    credo, 46–7
    developing personal qualities, 54–5
    empathy, 49–51
    essence, 46–7
    extra things, 31–2
    feedback, constructive, 61–5
    genuineness, 51–2
    person-centred theory, 48
    self-awareness, 55–60
    unconditional positive regard (UPR),
        53–4
support/challenge balance, clinical
    supervision, 79–82
supportive category, six-category
    intervention analysis, 109, 121–3

taking care of yourself, stress, 187–8
target, clinical supervision, 5–6
therapy, supervision, 8–10
training, clinical supervision, 21–2
transferable skills, 15–17

unconditional positive regard (UPR),
    supervision relationship, 53–4
understanding, listening skills, 102

valid interventions, six-category
    intervention analysis, 124–5

'why' questions
    listening skills, 95–6